Shiitake

Also by Kenneth Jones:

Pau d'Arco: Immune Power from the Rain Forest
Reishi: Ancient Herb for Modern Times

Shiitake

The Healing Mushroom

KENNETH JONES

Healing Arts Press
Rochester, Vermont

Healing Arts Press
One Park Street
Rochester, Vermont 05767

Note to the reader: *This book is intended as an informational guide. The remedies,
approaches, and techniques described herein are meant to supplement, and not to be a
substitute for, professional medical care or treatment. They should not be used to treat a
serious ailment without prior consultation with a qualified healthcare professional.*

Library of Congress Cataloging-in-Publication Data

Jones, Kenneth, 1954–
   Shiitake : the healing mushroom / by Kenneth Jones.
      p. cm.
   Includes bibliographical references and index.
   ISBN 978-0-89281-499-2
   1. Shiitake—Therapeutic use. I. Title.
RM666.S465J66 1994
615'.329222—dc20   94-1557
                                             CIP

Printed and bound in the United States

10 9 8 7 6 5 4

Interior design and layout by Bonnie Atwater
This book was typeset in Frutiger, with Italian Electric as a display face

Healing Arts Press is a division of Inner Traditions International

Distributed to the book trade in Canada by Publishers Group West (PGW), Toronto, Ontario

Distributed to the health food trade in Canada by Alive Books, Toronto and Vancouver

Distributed to the book trade in the United Kingdom by Deep Books, London

Distributed to the book trade in Australia by Millennium Books, Newtown, N. S. W.

Distributed to the book trade in New Zealand by Tandem Press, Auckland

Contents

Preface

I was five years into a jungle of studies on South American herbs and the immune system when the name *Lentinus edodes*, the Latin handle for a mushroom called shiitake (she-tah-key), began raising its head. The literature on botanical sources of immunostimulants was heavily infected with this fungus, and I didn't even know what it was. When finally I looked, it turned out to be a mushroom and an edible one at that. I was delighted to find that it had a flavor renowned all over the world, but most North Americans were in the dark about it. Now ten years later, and with the enormous demand for ethnic foods, the situation has changed. Articles on the mushroom have appeared in all the major health magazines, and the name shiitake is heard everywhere from sitcoms to the daily news.

When I began to see the wealth of research that had already been done on shiitake in Japan, more than for many medicinal plants, I couldn't believe my eyes. This great-tasting mushroom had shown considerable pharmacologic activity. Anyone who will take the time to look will see that shiitake demonstrates a fertile ground for the continual research of medicinal mushrooms worldwide. In fact, a surprising number of mushrooms used in folk medicine have demonstrated significant activity against disease. But once again, we Westerners have been the last ones to learn.

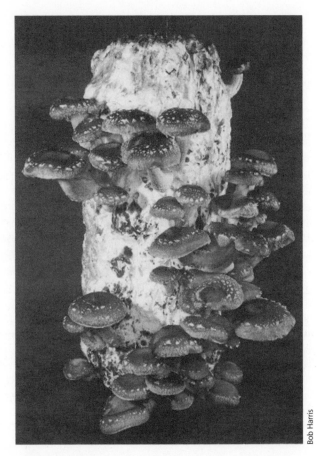

Completely overrun with shiitake mycelium, a sawdust log brings forth a harvest of fruit-bodies.

ONE

A Food from the Forest

In the Oriental marketplace, whether here or across the Pacific, the shiitake mushroom is one of the most cherished of foods. In Japan, where for centuries the best products were reserved for royalty, shiitake has been called the "king" or "monarch of the mushrooms," thereby denoting a food of superior taste and quality. *Shiitake* is a Japanese name deriving from *take*, mushroom, and *shii*, a kind of chestnut tree *(Castanopsis cuspidata)* that the mushroom was commonly found growing on in Japan.[1] As a forest mushroom, shiitake will grow on many kinds of trees, including alder, chestnut, maple, oak, walnut, and ebony.[2] When fresh, it has the coloration of a young fawn, complete with those lighter-colored spots. When dried, the cap becomes cracked, taking on the appearance of old leather.

The legacy of shiitake as a highly regarded food plant was furthered by the British botanist Miles Joseph Berkeley (1803–1889). He made certain that people would eventually notice its delights when he named it *Lentinus edodes*, the Latin *edodes* meaning edible.[3] Recently, shiitake's Latin name was changed to *Lentinula edodes* (Berkeley) Pegler, but that did nothing to affect its appeal. Next to the common table mushroom *(Agaricus bisporus)*, shiitake is the most popular and most cultivated of all exotic mushrooms worldwide.[4] Fresh or dried, in seasonings, sauces, soup mixes, noodle stocks, carbonated health drinks, food supplements, and candies, shiitake has about as many uses in the Oriental diet as tomatoes have in the West. One Japanese product uses the mushroom to produce a potassium-rich yogurt drink.[5] In North America, shiitake's versatility and caramel-like flavor have not gone unnoticed: shiitake dishes are turning up in premier restaurants and fine cuisine magazines.[6] But flavor is not the only reason this mushroom has come to be praised.

NUTRITIONAL VALUE

Shiitake's food value alone makes the mushroom a welcomed contribution to our increasingly diet-conscious world. Shiitake is a good source of protein, potassium, and, including the stems, zinc, an important element for immune competence. It is also a rich source of complex carbohydrates called polysaccharides and contains more than one that is known to potentiate the immune system, a subject we will take up in later chapters.

If all these factors seem a lot for one mushroom, that is not surprising; mushrooms are a neglected source of human nutrition. The director of the Research Centre for Food Protein at the Chinese University of Hong Kong, Professor S. T. Chang, states, "When one considers that they can be produced on waste materials—converting products of little or no market value into food for an over-populated world—then there is no doubt that mushrooms represent one of the world's greatest untapped resources of nutritious and palatable food for the future."[7]

How many know, for instance, that the proteins in mushrooms hold all the essential amino acids needed in our diet? Or that they contain generous amounts of leucine and lysine, essential amino acids found wanting in the majority of our cereals? Mushrooms are higher in essential amino acids than soybeans, kidney beans, peanuts, or corn. They place almost as high as milk.[8] Amino acids make up close to 14 percent of the dry shiitake mushroom,[9] and essential amino acids make up more than 40 percent of the amino acid content of shiitake's protein.[10] A study of Japanese adult males who ate 40 grams of the mushroom per day as part of a prescribed diet found a very high digestibility (85.5 ± 23.8 percent) of shiitake's protein.[11] Apart from shiitake, fresh mushrooms generally have about double the protein of vegetables and are low in calories. They are good sources of

Japanese indoor culture of shiitake with a floor of logs ready to fruit.

vitamins B_1 (thiamine) and B_2 (riboflavin), niacin, iron, and phosphorus. And when it comes to nucleic acids, the average in mushrooms (7.1 percent) is more than cereals (1.1–4 percent) or meats (2.2–5.7 percent).[12]

Ergosterol, a solid plant alcohol, is found in considerable quantities in dried shiitake.[13] If the mushroom receives adequate sunlight or irradiation with ultraviolet light, the ergosterol is convertible to vitamin D. The vitamin D in shiitake increased 2.5 times after only three hours of exposure to sunlight. In fact, shiitake is already higher in vitamin D than most foods. Some samples contain 56 international units (IU) per mushroom.[14] If shiitake is irradiated with sunlight, then as few as four or five dried mushrooms would equal the U.S. daily recommended allowance of 400 IU.[15] This is especially pertinent to vegetarians, since a number of studies have found them to be deficient in vitamin D.[16]

CULTIVATION

In China, shiitake is called *hsiang ku,* which means "fragrant mushroom," a fitting name in light of its caramel-like odor. In North America, shiitake, Chinese black mushroom, and Chinese forest mushroom are the names most commonly used. In the forests of China and Japan, shiitake still grows in the wild. With a name like forest mushrooms, some people expect that they can be gathered only in the woods. But, in fact, systems of cultivation were known in China as far back as the twelfth century,[17] and now reliable growing methods are available to anyone who wishes to grow them at home or commercially.[18]

Shiitake cultivation employs the enriched sawdust of hardwoods or the more traditional slower method of inoculating hardwood logs. Until this century, inoculation methods were largely reliant on luck. Basically, they consisted of smearing shiitake into cuts made in logs. As a student of agriculture at Kyoto University during the 1940s, Kisaku Mori witnessed the economic ruin of shiitake farmers who commonly called upon the help of Buddhist priests to make prayers, literally calling the mushrooms to grow. One day in Kyushu, he encountered a group of farmers who were faced with abandoning their village if the prayers of the priest failed. Moved by their plight, he determined to develop a reliable growing method,[19] and he did.

TABLE 1
NUTRITIONAL FACTORS

ELEMENTS IN DRIED SHIITAKE[20]	CAPS	STEMS
Copper (micrograms/gram: µg/g)	15.4	9.1
Iron (µg/g)	88.3	46.5
Zinc (µg/g)	–	83.0
Manganese (µg/g)	37.2	60.9
Nitrogen (milligrams/gram: mg/g)	37.5	14.3
Phosphorus (mg/g)	10.7	13.9
Potassium (mg/g)	33.9	27.3
Sodium (mg/g)	0.2	0.5
Calcium (mg/g)	0.2	0.6
Magnesium (mg/g)	1.9	3.8

GENERAL COMPONENTS OF FRESH SHIITAKE (%)[21]	CAPS	STEMS
Ash	0.9	0.6
Crude fat	0.2	0.1
Crude protein	1.9	1.7
Crude fiber	0.9	1.6
Saccharide	5.9	10.9

VITAMIN D IN SHIITAKE (IU/100 g)[22]	
Whole fresh:	
Outdoor cultured	390
Indoor cultured	73
Whole dried:	
Various culture methods	969

POLYSACCHARIDE CONTENT (DRIED SHIITAKE) (%)[23]	
Caps	38.3–39.5
Stems	48.7–51.6
Mycelium	53.5–59.3

NUTRITIONALLY ESSENTIAL AMINO ACIDS (g/100 g)	MYCELIUM[24]	FRUIT-BODY[25]
Arginine	1.25	7.0
Histidine	0.393	1.8
Leucine	1.92	7.0
Isoleucine	1.35	4.4
Lysine	0.799	3.5
Tyrosine	0.81	3.5
Threonine	0.978	5.2
Methionine	0.355	1.8
Phenylalanine	1.18	5.3
Valine	1.19	5.2

NUTRITIONALLY ESSENTIAL AMINO ACIDS (g/100 g)	DRIED FRUIT-BODY[26]	COOKED[26]
Arginine	0.648	0.089
Histidine	0.159	0.022
Leucine	0.679	0.093
Isoleucine	0.405	0.055
Lysine	0.343	0.047
Tyrosine	0.323	0.044
Threonine	0.497	0.068
Methionine	0.179	0.025
Phenylalanine	0.486	0.067
Tryptophan	0.031	0.044
Valine	0.486	0.067

PROTEIN (%)[27]	DRIED FRUIT-BODY
	17.5

FATTY ACID CONTENT: SHIITAKE CAPS (g/100g)[28]	DRIED	COOKED
Monounsaturated fatty acids	0.307	0.140
Polyunsaturated fatty acids	0.140	0.031
Saturated fatty acids	0.247	0.055

Wood plugs colonized with shiitake mycelium—a stringy white vegetative matter that develops to become cap and stem—are fitted into holes drilled in the logs. The holes are then covered with wax, and the logs are hammered or vibrated from time to time to stimulate mycelial growth,[29, 30] a practice known since at least the fourteenth century, when logs were beaten with a club to "wake up" the mushroom.[31] Under the right conditions of moisture and temperature, the mushrooms crop up from the mycelium, producing their stems and caps. After one to two years, the logs, now permeated with the mycelium, will send forth the harvest each year in the fall and spring for another three and sometimes five years.[32] Another method uses synthetic logs made of sawdust, millet, and wheat bran. They can yield four times the harvest of natural logs in a tenth of the time.[33]

As food supplements, various shiitake products are now widely available in health food stores. Most dried shiitake is imported from China and Japan, and you can buy it by the sackful in Oriental food markets everywhere in North America. Prices vary, depending on the fullness of the cap: usually, the fuller the cap, the better the flavor. In Japan, the thinner-capped shiitake are called *koshin,* and the fuller-capped are called *donko* shiitake.

Shiitake has long been Japan's largest agricultural export, but there are increasing numbers of shiitake growers in North America; well over one thousand cultivators—the majority growing the mushroom in their homes—are actively engaged at every level of production.[34] By 1987 shiitake had become the most widely cultivated specialty mushroom in the United States, making up over 66 percent of the market.[35] By the late 1990s, U.S. shiitake production could become a major industry.[36] In 1990–91, domestic production had already reached 3,900,000 pounds.[37] But these figures are not as dramatic as one might think: worldwide, shiitake production accounts for 14 percent of all mushrooms grown.[38]

For those interested in becoming growers on any level, a number of excellent books on shiitake cultivation are now available in English. Topping my list are *Shiitake Grower's Handbook* by Paul Przybillowicz and J. Donaghue (Kendall Hunt Publishing Co., Dubuque, Iowa, 1991), *Growing Gourmet and Medicinal Mushrooms* by Paul Stamets (Ten Speed Press,

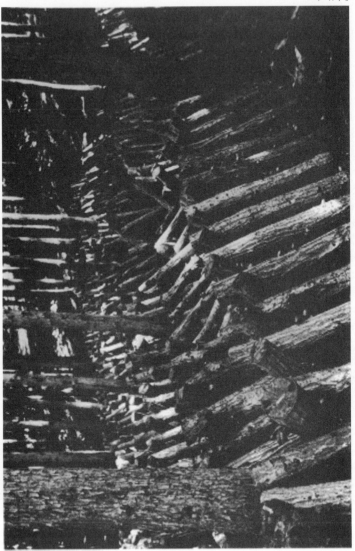

Shiitake fruiting on stacked logs in a Japanese forest.

Berkeley, Calif., 1993), and *Growing Shiitake Commercially* by Bob Harris (The Second Foundation Publications, Summertown, Tenn., 1993).

The average amount of all mushrooms consumed per person in the United States during the 1960s was 6 ounces (oz) per year. By 1989 that figure had grown to 36 oz per year.[39] In the chapters ahead, we will see that whether people use shiitake to help lower cholesterol, to strengthen the immune system, or as a source of valuable compounds for medical research, the potential of this mushroom extends well beyond the realm of culinary delights.

SHIITAKE RECIPES

Gourmets rave about shiitake. Scarcely any Oriental cookbook today can be found without at least one recipe for the mushroom, and the health benefits make them all the more enticing at the table. Try some of these recipes and find out for yourself.

Sweet Black Forest Mushroom

From Kay Shimizu's *Cooking with Exotic Mushrooms* (Tokyo: Shufunotomo Co., 1977).

10 large dried shiitake, reconstituted in 2 cups warm water; cover for 15 minutes

1/2 tablespoon sugar

1/4 teaspoon salt

2 teaspoons light soy sauce

1 tablespoon mirin (sweet rice cooking wine)

After soaking shiitake, trim off the heavy stems. Cut the caps if desired into pie-shaped wedges. Pour off the top of the mushroom-soaking liquid into a saucepan, discarding the sediment remaining at the bottom. Boil shiitake with the sugar in the liquid for 5 minutes. Add salt and soy sauce. Simmer another 5 minutes. Add mirin a minute before removing from stove. Allow shiitake to soak for 10–15 more minutes to accumulate as much additional flavor and juice as possible. Remove to a dish and serve at room temperature. This is particularly good as a side dish for dinner or as an addition to a Japanese picnic lunch. Serves two or more, as long as the guests don't get greedy.

Shiitake Sweet and Sour Salad

From *Shiitake News*, March 1993, p. 12.

½ cup fresh shiitake

1 garlic clove, minced

½ cup onion rings

¼ cup herb salad dressing

2 cups fresh green vegetables

Mix the shiitake, garlic, onion rings, and dressing, and sauté until the onion rings are tender. Add the whole mixture to salad greens. Toss and serve. Provides two servings.

Shiitake and Prawns

From the author's kitchen.

16 dried shiitake caps

3 garlic cloves

3 tablespoons butter, melted

1 handful of pea pods

2 packages of Chinese instant noodles (without seasoning)

1 pound shelled prawns or jumbo shrimp

3 tablespoons teriyaki sauce

Soak the mushroom caps in warm water for 15 minutes. Squeeze out the water by hand, saving the shiitake-water for later. Cut the caps into strips and remove the tough centers. Crush the garlic and add it to the melted butter.

Set a frying pan or wok over medium high heat. Steam the pea pods or sauté them in garlic butter, and prepare the noodles as instructed on the package. Separately sauté the prawns in garlic butter until cooked (when they turn a lighter color). Add the pea pods, the soaked shiitake strips, and the teriyaki sauce as desired. Add a splash or two of the shiitake-water and cover for 30 seconds to finish. To serve, place the noodles on a plate and top them with shiitake and prawns. Serves two very hungry people or three as a side dish.

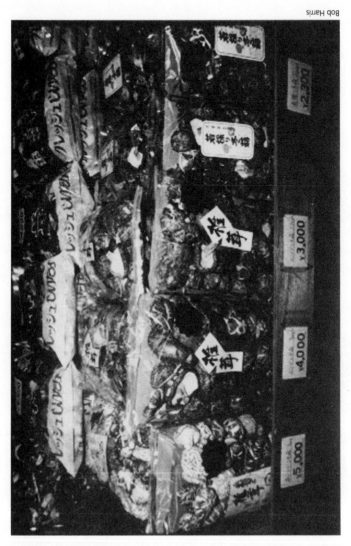

Various grades of dried shiitake sold in Japan.

TWO

Shiitake in Folk Medicine

In Oriental folk medicine, shiitake is a food that *activates* the blood. As simple as that sounds, the mushroom is used for a remarkable array of health problems. It is indicated in folk treatments of colds, measles in children, bronchial inflammation, stomachache, headache, faintness, dropsy (fluid accumulation in tissues), smallpox, and mushroom poisoning.[1]

Added to these older traditional uses, in Japan there are modern-day accounts of high blood pressure normalizing or being substantially lowered from eating eight mushrooms a day for a couple of weeks. In view of some of the latest research on shiitake in heart disease, a subject taken up in the next chapter, anecdotal accounts like these are no longer surprising. Others have reported the mushroom of benefit in such diverse problems as ulcers, gout, low blood pressure, constipation, myopia, poor vision, allergies, hemorrhoids, pyorrhea, neuralgia (pain along nerves), poor complexion, and sexual weakness.[2]

Uses of the mycelial extract of shiitake are very similar to those of the fruit-body. For example, there are preparations of the mycelium for the bath to enhance the beauty of the skin[3] and one for dermatological diseases that clinical tests found efficacious in the treatment of skin rash and acne.[4] Cases recorded from clinical and anecdotal settings in Japan are numerous. Patients and physicians have reported the mycelial extract effective against stomach ulcer, cirrhosis, hepatitis B, liver infection, diabetes, leukemia, hypertension (high blood pressure), rheumatism, allergies (including allergic asthma), and autoimmune diseases such as purpura,[5, 6] which is attended by an itchy, reddish purple rash.

It is recorded that in ancient times members of the Japanese courts regarded shiitake as an aphrodisiac and defended the growing sites by keeping them hidden and well guarded. History also tells us that the emperors of China ate the mushroom in great quantities to slow the onset of old age.[7] Today, shiitake is among the foods and herbal medicines in the Chinese diet that nutritionists have determined are rich in "anti-aging activities." For that reason, shiitake was recently listed by the Chinese Academy of Medical Sciences as a promising candidate for research devoted to caring for the rapidly growing segment of China's population aged sixty and over. By 2025 the number in that age group will have reached an estimated 208,000,000 people.[8]

In China during the Ming dynasty (A.D. 1368–1644), shiitake was already recognized as a medicinal food. In an extensive interview by the Tokyo magazine *Sejikai* (*Political World*, September 1981), Professor Chiyokichi Iizuka, Ph.D., of Tsukuba University related the notes of a famous doctor from that era named Gorin,[9] or Wu Rui.[10] In 1309 he wrote the *Materia Medica for Daily Use*.[11] As translated into Japanese, Wu wrote, "*Shiitake wa ki o eki shi, vezu, kaze o naoshi, chi o yaburu*," meaning that shiitake improves "ki [or *chi*, meaning spirit or vital energy], doesn't starve, cures cold, and penetrates into the blood circulatory system." Iizuka explained that more accurately, this means shiitake makes one more "lively." The mushroom increases "vital energy," which in today's terminology would mean that it increases stamina,[12] or that "shiitake can endow people with vigor and energy."[13]

In traditional Chinese medicine, shiitake is categorized as a food that has an "upward" effect upon the "yang" energy of the body and corresponds to a "sweet" flavor with a "neutral" energy. The organ given as corresponding to shiitake is the stomach. Foods classified as sweet are said to act on the spleen and stomach and are used to slow acute symptoms and to neutralize the toxic actions of foods. Sweet foods are recommended in cases in which the digestive system is weak. The upward movement category for shiitake means that it would generally be used to treat ailments of the lower body, such as a prolapsed uterus, gastroptosis (falling stomach), or diarrhea.[14]

Wu Rui was very specific in stating that shiitake is "good for treatment of Heart Troubles . . . beneficial to [all forms of] Malignancy, likewise certainly [good for] Snake's Poison, Tapeworms, the One Inch Whiteworms, and all manner of [intestinal] worms." Nearly seven centuries later, there are strong pharmacological bases for the use of shiitake in heart troubles and malignancies; both are subjects we will explore in later chapters. Wu also wrote that shiitake fought "Hunger" and belonged to a class of medicines that "breaks up" blood.[15] Further to this matter, Iizuka added that shiitake "banishes bad blood or purifies blood that is slightly acidic; that is to say it makes the blood alkaline . . . improves the flow of blood . . . makes the blood flow to the very end of the capillary vessels [smallest blood vessels]."[16] Wu had also noted that it was effective in preventing and treating what we now know to be cerebral hemorrhage.[17]

Whereas the Ming dynasty doctor had referred to shiitake "curing cold," the term for this action is *shinkeishokanja* (rheumatic patients). Iizuka noted that "curing cold" has the same meaning as *gofu* in the phrase *kampo ni gofu ari* (Chinese medicine takes care of five-evil wind). While the traditional Chinese medical concept of a *cold* condition would imply migraines, strokes, arthritis, the common cold, and epilepsy, he hastened to explain that in old China, arthritis (*tong feng*) was what we would now call chronic joint rheumatism. As for epilepsy, he admitted the clinical proof was missing; however, he knew an authority on traditional Chinese medicine who had written that shiitake decoction (simmered in water) is effective against this malady.[18] Today, a number of physicians tell me that what he refers to as "chronic joint rheumatism" may well be fibromyalgia syndrome, the so-called lesser cousin of chronic fatigue syndrome (CFS). Shiitake is already playing a major role in the treatment of CFS, and many of those patients suffer from both syndromes. We will return to that important subject in a later chapter.

THE MUSHROOM AND THE FLU

On the surface, the various diseases that shiitake is reputed to alleviate are numerous enough to lead us to think the mushroom might be some kind of cure-all. But as more and more research has inadvertently shown, many of the folk applications do have some basis in fact; in some instances, a very strong basis. The cold is one example.

Contemporary cases of colds being "cured" when shiitake is taken are reportedly numerous in Japan.[19] According to the late Kisaku Mori, former head of the Mushroom Research Institute of Japan, shiitake was regarded as a cure for colds during the Ming dynasty some six hundred years ago.[20] But it wasn't until the 1960s that medical researchers began to ask why.

As early as 1966, Kenneth W. Cochran and colleagues at the University of Michigan at Ann Arbor discovered that shiitake could produce a highly significant level of protection against a type A influenza. Type A flu viruses are the ones that create major outbreaks and can become epidemic and even pandemic, spreading from continent to continent. With the injection of a "crude" mushroom extract, the average number of lung lesions in mice in the wake of flu infection decreased by 46 percent. The clinically proven anti-influenza drug amantadine hydrochloride produced a comparable 40 percent score.[21]

Later evidence showed the anti-influenza action could partly be attributed to shiitake's spores. Made up into a water extract, the spores proved more active than the mushroom.[22] Besides the stem and cap, in smaller amounts, the particle-sized spores also showed up in the mycelium, even after heat treatment to 33 degrees C. (91 degrees F.). This research was taken deeper when the active part of the spores was isolated and it was found that they held, of all things, "virus-like particles" similar in structure to an influenza virus.[23] The discovery that these particles had induced the body's own production of interferon—a powerful protein component of the immune system that literally interferes with viral reproduction—and in amounts sufficient to protect against influenza, inspired much more intensive research. When extractives from the virus-like particles consisting of double-stranded RNA (ribonucleotide) were used, antitumor effects were found as well.[24, 25] The effect was stronger than that of an interferon-inducing drug known today as Ampligen (polyribonucleotide), but the spore products were never developed into a drug,[26] probably because the amount of interferon induced by Ampligen is four times that of the mushroom RNA.[27]

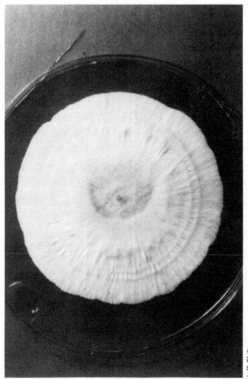

Mycelium growing in a petri dish.

At Tohoku University in Japan, a team led by Dr. Fujio Suzuki conducted more extensive experiments with shiitake RNA against type A influenza in the early 1970s. They found that if mice were given just one dose of the RNA (8 mg/kg) an hour before being infected with the flu intranasally, 60 percent survived. With the same dose of the anti-influenza drug amantadine given three hours before plus one hour before flu infection, and then an hour and three hours following infection, plus a daily dose for four days, only 18 percent of the mice survived.[28]

Was the mystery of the anti-influenza action of shiitake solved, or were there still other factors? This question was the subject of another early investigation by Yasuhiro Yamamura and Kenneth W. Cochran. From the fruit-body, they uncovered a new substance possessing "marked and selective activity against orthomyxoviruses." These are viruses that cause symptoms in the mucous membrane. The new substance, dubbed Ac2P, was a water-soluble polysaccharide, a complex sugar made up of many simple sugar molecules, and it produced a 60 percent inhibition of influenza. Although how Ac2P worked remained unknown, the researchers concluded that it may be an important contributing factor to the high degree of shiitake's activity against influenza.[29]

At the same time that clinical studies to prove or disprove shiitake's benefits against influenza in people are lacking, the folklore from China,[30] and apparently numerous cases reported in Japan, would have us believe that the treatment of colds was to some degree successful. So convinced was he of shiitake's efficacy against colds that Kisaku Mori, a world authority on the mushroom, urged the public to eat them for "the benefits they offer in curing colds," a therapeutic effect, he insisted, proven by "many case reports."[31] Of course, those million-dollar clinical studies to find out for sure still go begging, as they do for hundreds of unpatentable natural products.

Taking shiitake tea for the flu was of no benefit to me, but then I had a particularly virulent strain of Taiwanese flu. Shiitake is apparently not a cure-all for the flu, but with the studies to date, it would not be surprising if one day we learned that the mushroom was helpful against particular kinds of flu and colds.

DIABETES AND LIVER AILMENTS

In his writings on the health benefits of shiitake, Kisaku Mori included several other folk uses of the mushroom neglected in research. Until recently, these had remained enigmatic. Mori noted that a "broth" of shiitake stems was employed as a "cure" for liver ailments and diabetes by the ancient Chinese, and that the broth had frequently been used as an admixture for their herbal medicines "to increase their efficacy."[32] Use of the mushroom to treat liver ailments is definitely more than folklore. Shiitake accelerates the processing of cholesterol in the liver[33, 34] and has shown a "very significant" protective effect in the livers of rats that have been subjected to a liver-damaging chemical (acetaminophen).[35] An extract of the mycelium is active against liver cancer and liver cancer formation resulting from a carcinogen.[36] The extract provided liver cell protection from damage caused by an autoimmune reaction[37] and was very successful in clinical use against chronic hepatitis B in people: every patient was cured.[38]

As for diabetes, what with the recently large body of studies now indicating an immunological[39, 40] or viral[41, 42] disorder as a basis for this disease, shiitake deserves a closer look. It has already had some attention in this field in Japan.

The School of Medicine at Tohoku University in Sendai found that *lentinan,* a polysaccharide derived from the fruit-body of shiitake, effectively inhibited insulin-dependent diabetes mellitus from developing in mice.[43] The other kind of diabetes, known as non-insulin-dependent, or Type II diabetes, is characterized by excessively high levels of blood sugar due to insufficient metabolism of glycogen, often because of obesity. In this kind of diabetes, the mycelial extract showed activity. When rats with the disease were fed the extract in doses equivalent to 1.6 to 3.2 grams a day for people, production of insulin increased (and levels of cholesterol decreased).[44] This last observation has greater implications than most people would think. In type II diabetes, which is the most common type, half the patients are at high risk for heart disease, owing in part to abnormally high levels of LDL cholesterol. As a result, these patients are susceptible to arteriosclerosis—a man with diabetes at forty has the heart of a man in his sixties. Not surprisingly, they are at least twice more likely to die from cardiovascular disease than the general population.[45]

The big question is whether the mycelial extract will do the same for people. While clinical trials to find out are lacking, one volunteer who had recurring Type II diabetes tried it (1 gram a day) and found that sugar excretion in the urine and levels of sugar in the blood normalized.[46] Getting blood sugar levels closer to normal through diet and medication reduces complications of diabetes by, on average, 60 percent. The intensive monitoring required to achieve this, however, is still very costly.[47]

One of the questions remaining is why it was specifically a broth of the stems that the ancients used to amplify their medicines. Because shiitake stems are tough to chew, in cooking they are commonly discarded, as they are with many kinds of mushrooms. But their delectable caramel-like flavor might have been reason enough for the ancients to use them to make herbal formulas with the hope of improving the taste of some unpalatable brew. In any event, it seems that the stems noticeably increased the efficacy of medicines to which they were added. The reasons could be many, for the stems contain medicinally active substances found in the rest of the mushroom, substances we are about to explore.

SAFETY

Millions of people enjoy the mushroom every day without the slightest complaint. But true to almost any food, for some people there are going to be allergic reactions. Too much of the fruit-body extract or tea may cause temporary diarrhea, but the reaction is apparently not serious.[48] Naturally, when this happens, one has only to stop taking the mushroom for a time, or stop taking so much.

Out of forty patients with chronic hepatitis B who were treated with large doses of a mycelial extract (6 grams a day), only one complained of any so-called side effects. These were abdominal bloating and looser stools. The symptoms were so mild that no change was needed in the therapy.[49] Outside of ingesting shiitake, some mushroom workers who breath the spores without protective dust masks, and some who handle the fruit-body or mycelium, have experienced allergic reactions, but these are still the exception.[50-54]

PREPARATION

For use of the mushroom fruit-bodies in maintaining health, the amount of shiitake recommended to eat daily is 3 to 4 grams. Twice this amount is used to remedy ailments, and in that application the tea and extract are preferred.[55] Not only are extracts more convenient than having to cook the mushroom, some are concentrated to provide ten times the amount of mushroom you get in a simple powdered mushroom product.

To make the medicinal decoction by the traditional method, begin by

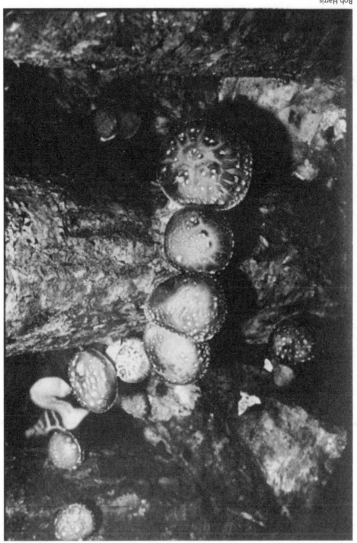

Shiitake fruiting on logs previously spiked with wooden plugs soaked in the mycelium.

drying fresh shiitakes under the sun (shiitake can be purchased already dried), then place them in a small amount of water (enough to cover), allow them to swell for 15 minutes or longer, and finally slice them for simmering. The tea is made using about a cup of hot water in which two sliced mushrooms are steeped.[56] Allow them to steep for half an hour, or, better still, about 20 minutes over low heat (not hot enough to make the water boil). Simmering for roughly half an hour will deplete the water, so that more will have to be added. Generally, twice the volume of the pre-soaked mushrooms is enough water for a short decoction. Grinding the mushrooms into a powder or chopping them into small pieces naturally increases the availability of active constituents in the decoction. The remainder can be removed by straining the brew while pouring and can be saved for cooking or fertilizer.

TABLE 2

USES OF SHIITAKE IN TRADITIONAL CHINESE MEDICINE[57]

General health maintenance	3 to 4 grams of mushroom a day
Mushroom poisoning	9 grams dried shiitake cooked in water; broth taken in one day
Measles in children	6 grams of dried shiitake simmered in water; broth taken twice daily
Stomachache	9 grams dried shiitake simmered in water; taken daily
Headaches and faintness	Cooked shiitake eaten daily; amount according to need
High cholesterol or atherosclerosis	9 grams dried or 90 grams fresh shiitake daily; powdered in capsules or cooked
High blood pressure	8 mushrooms a day
Liver ailments or diabetes	8 mushrooms a day
Flus and colds	6 to 8 grams shiitake made into a tea or extract

THREE

Shiitake and Cholesterol

Japan now has a major health problem in common with North America and Europe, and it is probably from adopting a more Western-style diet. Both the cure and the prevention of hardening of the arteries number among the most crucial problems identified by Japanese health authorities. Indeed, about half the deaths in Japan in the aged and middle-aged are due to some form of "hardening of the blood vessels."[1]

Atherosclerosis develops when the flow of blood in arteries becomes blocked by cholesterol-containing plaques called *atheroma*. Most authorities on heart disease believe we could increase our chances of survival by some means of reducing the daily amount of stress in our lives as well as the excessive fat in our blood.

How can shiitake help? Shiitake inhibits the aggregation or clumping together of blood platelets.[2] By inhibiting blood platelets from forming clots, which can lead to heart attacks, the mushroom fills the role of a blood tonic for the heart.

THE SECRET OF SLUDGE

Finding that mushrooms contain appreciable amounts of aggregation-inhibitory substances led Dr. Y. Hokama of the University of Hawaii at Manoa to take a closer look. In 1981 he partly identified these substances as derivatives of nucleic acid and discovered a very high yield (25.5 percent) in a water extract of shiitake.[3]

The topic of aggregated blood appeared in the West shortly after World War II. At the University of Chicago, Dr. Melvin H. Knisely called it a

23

"circulating mass of agglutinated cells," or "sludged blood." He didn't arrive at this name lightly. Two other universities had collaborated on a massive military project to study the effects of malaria on the blood. Having compared the behavior of blood in normal, healthy subjects with the blood of unhealthy people, in 1947 they presented an outline of sixteen years of research. What they ended up with was evidence of an overlooked perspective of blood in the mainstream of Western medicine: sticky masses of agglutinated red blood cells were found in association with a remarkable array of diseases but not in healthy subjects.[4]

To name some of the more familiar diseases, they found this changed blood in patients with malaria, fever, rheumatic fever (acute), rheumatoid arthritis, thrombotic purpura, hysteria, acute alcoholism, traumatic shock, measles, smallpox, whooping cough, scarlet fever, typhoid fever, diptheria, syphilis, chronic lymphatic leukemia, myologous leukemia, cancer (pancreas, esophagus, and colon), varicose ulcers, multiple sclerosis, sickle cell anemia, pneumonia, lung abscesses, the common cold, bronchitis, nephritis, malignant hypertension, arteriosclerotic heart disease, and pericarditis, a disease in which the sac surrounding the heart becomes inflamed.[5]

It may be no coincidence that nearly half of these diseases are found in folk and popular uses of shiitake, or that in folk medicine the mushroom was specifically thought of as a food used to activate the "blood circulatory system"[6] and to prevent or even treat "cerebral hemorrhage."[7]

Recent studies have shown that levels of aggregated blood, or highly viscous (sticky) blood, are higher in people with high blood pressure who also have enlarged hearts (left ventricle enlargement) than in those who simply have high blood pressure. Because patients with enlarged left ventricles are far more likely to die from a heart attack,[8] lowering their blood viscosity could be an inexpensive preventive measure. But don't hold your breath. Since at least 1957, coronary artery disease patients have been noted to have aggregated red blood cells and a reduced flow of blood, especially following a meal high in fats.[9] In 1988, Swiss scientists reported cholesterol-sensitive blood platelets in patients with high blood pressure, or hypertension, compared to subjects without it. They found this with low-density lipoprotein, or the LDL cholesterol we hear so much about in the daily news. In hypertensive patients, more LDL cholesterol caused blood platelets to aggregate in parallel with increases in blood pressure.[10]

Obviously, for some people cholesterol plays a significant role in creating these sludges in the first place. But after about the age of thirty, the walls of our blood vessels don't relax as much, and that leads to platelets sticking together, or aggregating. With reduced blood vessel relaxation, blood flow is decreased, and flushing out the sludges is impaired. Worse yet, the sludges have an even better chance of sticking to the walls of our arteries when we are stressed, and their chances improve again from diets rich in cholesterol.

Arterial risk factors such as high blood pressure, high levels of fats in the blood (hyperlipidemia), and diabetes are associated with impotence. When two or more of these factors are present, arteriosclerotic lesions in the arteries of the penis may be suspected. In Western medicine, such patients are advised to adhere to treatments otherwise prescribed for more serious hardening of the arteries (arteriosclerosis).[11] That shiitake was "highly regarded" as an aphrodisiac[12] by the ancients[13] and has definite anti-arteriosclerotic activity has not gone unnoticed.[14] If there is any basis for a sexually restorative property to the mushroom, this action appears the most likely cause.[15, 16] Some investigators believe zinc levels in the fruit-body of shiitake may be responsible for both the purported longevity and aphrodisiac effects; however, quantities of zinc in shiitake can vary greatly.[17]

MUSHROOMS AND THE HEART

The health-promoting action of mushrooms became the focus of a study in the USSR in 1988. Dr. Li Hwa Ryong and colleagues at the USSR Cardiology Research Center and the Institute of Nutrition of the Academy of Medical Sciences in Moscow teamed up to determine the potential of edible mushrooms against heart disease.[18, 19] They found thirteen of twenty different mushrooms were active against the formation of cholesterol-containing plaques (atheroma). Of these, nine showed anti-atherogenic activity as well: not only did they inhibit cholesterol build-up, but they also inhibited the formation of the resulting lesions so common in the arteries of heart disease patients. These lesions are formed of thick, degenerated tissue on the innermost part of the arterial wall.[20] Besides shiitake, three Oriental varieties had noteworthy levels of action: matsutake mushroom (*Armillaria matsutake*), kootake mushroom (*Sarcodon aspratus*), and the reishi mushroom (*Ganoderma lucidum*),[21] a "mushroom of longevity" in traditional Chinese medicine, used to increase the defenses or boost the chi (spirit or life energy), which the Japanese call *ki*.[22, 23] As noted in the last chapter, shiitake is also a ki tonic, one that fourteenth-century physician Wu Rui claimed was "good for treatment of Heart Troubles."[24] Over six hundred years later, science is beginning to find some weight to this bit of folklore.

The next step of Dr. Ryong was to determine the effect of the most active mushrooms. He discovered that the mushrooms had so thoroughly permeated the system that samples of blood serum (the clear part with red cells removed) from healthy people, who after a short fast had eaten a single dose (120 grams in this case) of the more active mushrooms and nothing else, significantly decreased the level of cholesterol in atherosclerotic cells taken from their unhealthy patients.[25]

In the end, only two mushrooms were selected as single-dose "dietary supplements" for tests in chronic heart disease patients. These were the shiitake mushroom and a powdered alcoholic extract (1.5 grams) of the reishi mushroom, the most active of all the mushrooms tested. Remarkably, the blood serum of these chronic heart disease patients had a toxic influence on cultures of healthy heart cells, causing cholesterol to accumulate and atheroma to form. But that changed after taking either mushroom. The results were very significant: as long as five hours after a single meal of shiitake, or a single dose in the case of reishi, the once toxic blood serum had "lost the ability to cause cholesterol accumulation" by 30 to 41 percent.[26]

There are also signs that shiitake may help in *directly* alleviating high blood pressure. It suppressed high blood pressure in hypertensive rats that fed on the mushroom powder. Significant benefits were apparent after only fourteen days.[27] This effect is also true of the reishi mushroom and has been demonstrated clinically in people.[28, 29]

Pilot studies with heart disease patients in China found high blood pressure and high cholesterol were significantly improved with reishi in 20 to

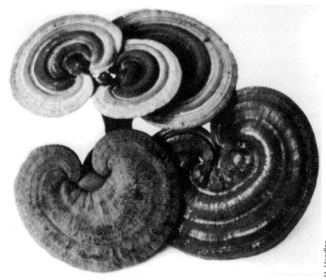

Reishi mushrooms

48 percent of cases. Cholesterol levels dropped in 68 percent of cases after a few months on the mushroom extract (3 to 6 grams/day).[30] Studies from seven hospitals in China show general improvements in heart disease reached 81.77 percent of cases.[31] Because their activities are demonstrably similar, herbalists here are using reishi and shiitake extracts combined to complement their actions.

The reishi mushroom has been the subject of intensive research in the Orient for many years.[32] Besides heart disease, some North American doctors are applying reishi against chronic fatigue syndrome, autoimmune disorders, and cancer. More than one Canadian doctor has found reishi to be a "clinically effective tonic," but it is one for which controlled clinical studies are still lacking.[33]

STUDIES IN JAPAN

In the search for foods to prevent heart attacks, shiitake is one with three possible benefits: inhibiting the formation of sludged or aggregated blood;

reducing the level of cholesterol; and lowering high blood pressure.[34]

Early investigations of shiitake against cholesterol were initiated to determine the real, if any, benefits this long-held "elixir of life" could offer to the people of Japan. If feeding studies were any indication, even with rats, here was something of definite value. At Tohoku University the Department of Food Chemistry determined that the ground-up dried mushroom as 5 percent of the diet produced a marked reduction in blood levels of cholesterol. But rats on a diet of shiitake plus 1 percent cholesterol still had higher levels of cholesterol in their livers.[35] What was happening? A cholesterol-reducing amino acid in the mushroom called *eritadenine* was accelerating the rate at which cholesterol was being metabolized in the system,[36] thus the temporarily higher levels in the liver.

Shiitake accelerates the normal excretion of cholesterol into the feces by way of the liver. It is in the liver that cholesterol is processed for use by the body in its manufacture of bile acids and of steroid hormones. Before cholesterol leaves the liver to enter the blood, shiitake accelerates the conversion of so-called bad cholesterol (low-density lipoproteins or LDLs) into a form known as high-density lipoproteins or HDLs that actually contribute to lower levels of LDLs.[37] Put another way, shiitake reduces the level of the LDLs while at the same time allowing the good cholesterol (HDLs) to remain. In more recent times, very low-density lipoproteins (VLDLs), the precursors to LDLs, have come to be regarded as the underlying foe: the more VLDLs, the more the liver will produce the LDL form. However, shiitake lowers that type of cholesterol, too. In rats that have a gene defect giving them high blood pressure as they age, a diet containing 5 percent shiitake powder caused the VLDLs in their plasma to drop by 60 percent.[38]

Part of the cholesterol-lowering action of shiitake is attributable to fiber. The total dietary fiber content of the dried mushroom is about 37 to 46 percent. In fact, mushrooms are an even better source of dietary fiber than wild vegetables, which average around 27 percent total dietary fiber. Mushrooms average around 39 percent.[39]

When rats were fed a high-cholesterol diet containing isolated shiitake fiber (5 percent) devoid of the cholesterol-lowering amino acid eritadenine, total plasma cholesterol levels fell to 77 percent of those without the fiber in their feed. As might be expected, there was also a tendency for HDL cholesterol to increase. Even so, whole shiitake powder in their diet produced the best results: plasma cholesterol fell to 54 percent of the level of the controls (those without any shiitake product in their feed).[40]

Long-term feeding studies of mice demonstrated that shiitake's effect on cholesterol metabolism is undiminished so long as intake is maintained. One study found no indications that the metabolism would change to negate the cholesterol-lowering effect for at least half a lifetime, nor was there any indication it would stop after that. These and other studies also found that the health of the animals remained good, and that they weighed less than mice on ordinary feed that wasn't supplemented with fat. I calculate the equivalent difference for a person weighing about 175 pounds would be roughly eight to twelve pounds (lb).[41]

If it were not for the fact that shiitake isn't the only edible mushroom scientists have seen produce an inhibiting effect on body weight, that would be more easily discounted. As incredulous as this may seem, the Yamaguchi Women's College in Japan found that a gourmet mushroom called maitake (*Grifola frondosa*) had a similar effect in rats that were fattened with a diet high in both cholesterol and fat. Averaging 350 grams, the rats were then given either a normal diet or a diet with 5 percent consisting of maitake powder. Unheated, dry mushroom powder worked best. Over a period of eighteen weeks, rats without the powder in their feed continued to gain about forty grams of weight, whereas those with the unheated mushroom powder in their feed weighed about 40 grams less than their starting weight after the same period. For a 350-gram rat, that's a big loss.[42] (Eating the cooked mushroom to obtain this effect requires low heat.[43, 44] If the powder was heated in water to 122 degrees F., the amount of weight lost by the rats was diminished by 20 percent. At 140 degrees the weight loss diminished by 80 percent, and at 212 degrees there was no weight loss at all.[45] Whether the weight loss factor in shiitake is also affected by heat is not yet known.)

A pilot study at a Tokyo clinic with thirty overweight people on the mushroom found they lost from 6.6 to as much as 26.4 lb in eight weeks. Masanori Yokota, M.D., of the Koseikai Clinic in Tokyo, explained that the dose was 20 tablets of maitake a day, equivalent to 200 grams of fresh maitake. Except for the addition of maitake, the subjects made no change to their regular diet.[46]

Maitake grows wild in eastern Canada and the United States, where it occurs in grayish brown clusters as big as twenty inches wide at the base of deciduous and conifer trees and on stumps. A single cluster of these spoon-shaped caps can weigh as much as 100 lb.[47] The dried mushroom has a smoky-gray color and the appearance of tree lichen. Cooked, it is rich, even nutty in flavor, a lot like Cornish game hen. The only precaution for eating maitake is that owing to an unknown factor in the raw mushroom that destroys thiamine (vitamin B[1]), ideally maitake should be cooked before eating. To deactivate this thiaminase factor, the cooking temperature must exceed 158 degrees F.[48] But this factor is not something to worry about in the West, where the daily thiamine intake from food would alleviate the thiamine losses caused by maitake.

CLINICAL RESEARCH

In experiments with people consuming shiitake, the National Institute of Nutrition in Tokyo obtained results showing a substantial reduction in cholesterol. Somewhat better results were found in the young,[49] but there is no longer any doubt that shiitake could be of enormous benefit in reducing heart disease in all ages.

After only seven days, thirty "healthy young women" showed a decrease of serum cholesterol averaging 7 percent from eating the dried mushroom, which is soaked in water before cooking. From eating the fresh mushroom, they had an average 12 percent drop in cholesterol. Twenty women had eaten dried shiitake (9 grams a day) and ten had eaten an equivalent amount of fresh shiitake (90 grams a day). With the same number of participants, the results in people aged sixty or older revealed an average 9 percent decrease in serum cholesterol whether the mushrooms were dried or fresh.[50]

There were similar findings in a larger study with 420 young women and 40 elderly people. They ate the same amounts of the dried and fresh product daily as in the previous study. This time, however, the decrease in cholesterol after seven days was slightly greater in the elderly, showing a 7 to 15 percent drop, while readings in the young women ranged from 6 to 12 percent.[51]

Because the consumption of pork and sukiyaki is so common in Japan, one of the institute's scientists, Dr. Shinjiro Suzuki wondered what would happen to cholesterol levels in people eating shiitake when, as part of their diet, they also consumed a substantial amount of animal fat, the main source of excessive cholesterol. To find out, he recruited a group of young women and divided them into three groups of ten. One group added fresh shiitake (90 grams) to their diet; another added an equal amount of fresh shiitake and in addition consumed 60 grams of butter daily; a third group simply added the butter to their diet without any shiitake. After a week on these regimens, serum cholesterol levels for the first group fell within the predicted drop of the previous study results. For those who simply added butter to their diet—without the benefit of shiitake—there was a 14 percent increase in cholesterol. And for the group on shiitake plus 60 grams of butter a day, blood serum showed a decrease in cholesterol of 4 percent.[52]

Suzuki concluded that the addition of the mushroom to the diet had completely obviated the effect of the butter in raising cholesterol. The change in cholesterol levels with shiitake and the added butter in the diet represented an 18 percent drop! He suggests that in addition to enhancing the flavor of dishes rich in animal fats, shiitake may well be a preventive or even a "cure" for hardening of the arteries, a condition responsible for roughly half the deaths in Japan in the aged and middle-aged.[53]

A major study of cholesterol and heart disease published in 1986 indicates that every time we lower our cholesterol levels by 1 percent, the risk of heart disease, barring other factors, drops by 2 percent. For middle-aged men, about half of all deaths from heart disease are from too much cholesterol. Their risk of coronary heart disease increases with every increase in cholesterol.[54] For women the rate is lower, but at an average of 31 percent worldwide, it is still high.[55] The majority of people with excessive cholesterol need to get their levels down by 30 to 50 percent. There are drugs that will do this, but at what cost? An increase in the use of drugs usually spells increased side effects. And drugs are a pricey approach to a problem that for most can be remedied with changes to the diet. The Japanese diet, consisting mainly of carbohydrates and low in fats, is an often cited example of a better model for us to follow. Their coronary heart disease rates have been fairly low,[56] at least until recently.

The risk of certain kinds of cancer from high levels of cholesterol is something most people don't think of when cholesterol comes up, but it is being watched. From 1985 to 1987, Dutch investigators noticed a significantly higher incidence of breast cancer in those women who consumed more fat, no matter the source. Their data suggested that if women reduced their daily intake of fat to 30 percent of total food intake from the current 40 percent, the incidence of breast cancer might drop by 10 to 30 percent.[57]

In the spring of 1993, the release of a five-year study of lung cancer rates in American women carried some very disturbing news for hamburger lovers. The U.S. National Cancer Institute reported that for nonsmoking women who had diets with a high content of saturated fat, the risk of lung cancer was four times higher than average.[58]

The lungs rely on cells of the immune system, particularly macrophages, to clean up any foreign cells that might lead to tumors. And, yes, there are studies showing an impaired scavenging ability of macrophages and related immune cells as the result of high amounts of cholesterol in the diets of animals.[59] Why this area of diet and disease hasn't received greater attention is incomprehensible to me. Although these studies go back even earlier, in 1968 a team at the New York University School of Medicine reported that following the oral administration of digestible fats in mice, they had found a "prolonged depression" of the ability of macrophages to scavenge foreign cells.[60]

The U.S. Army made similar findings in monkeys. Given a diet high in fats and cholesterol, antibody development in the monkeys was impaired. The army doctors concluded that "altered immune function could contribute to the impaired host resistance that is said to be associated with an excess of body fat or dietary lipid intake." They advised that an "effort be made to evaluate the magnitude and importance of these relationships in man."[61]

Others have made the same kinds of observations, finding that a diet high in LDL cholesterol inhibits macrophages by clogging up their membranes.[62, 63] One team found a greater susceptibility to viral and bacterial infections in animals with high levels of cholesterol in their blood.[64] Because the macrophage, when activated, will also go after viruses and kill tumor cells, foods that lower cholesterol may turn out to be our best defense against the diseases now killing us in the greatest numbers.

FOUR

Cancer Research

Helping the body mount an immune cell attack against disease is today a practical reality called immunotherapy. As in other treatment approaches, the real hero is the body. With a supporting crew of specialized cells that make up the immune system, the body can ward off cancer cells, bacteria, viruses, and pathogenic fungi. Among the main characters of this system are the macrophages and T-lymphocytes, or T-cells, and these are the main immune cells that shiitake stimulates.

If sufficiently stimulated, T-cells are able to activate macrophages. Polysaccharides on the surface of bacteria also activate macrophages, and that is one way that polysaccharide-containing mushrooms can boost immunologic responses, essentially by mimicking foreign cells.

Polysaccharides are found throughout nature. They are made up of many units of sugar and form part of plant fiber. Some are commonly added to our foods as stabilizers and thickeners, such as guar gum and gum arabic. Experiments have shown that some polysaccharide sources in our diet may be playing a nutritional role, helping us to keep cholesterol levels down and helping diabetics with their glucose tolerance.[1] At the same time, many immune-system–modulating, especially "immunostimulating," polysaccharides have been discovered in mushrooms, particularly those used in Oriental folk medicine.[2, 3] Those in shiitake are of a type known as *beta*-glucans, which are typical of the immunoactive kind found in mushrooms.

In the fall of 1925, the respected British medical journal *The Lancet* carried an editorial suggesting that "medicinal properties attributed by tradition to certain species of fungi may possibly represent an untapped source of therapeutic virtue."[4] Nowhere has this possibility been explored with more success than in the laboratories and clinics of China and Japan. In traditional Chinese medicine fungi possess a wide range of immunological effects, enough, one might say, to call them pharmafoodicals. Currently, at least eighteen different commonly prescribed Chinese medicinal plants are known to contain immunomodulators of the polysaccharide kind.[5] Many studies of these complex sugars concern mushrooms used against cancer in folk medicine, one of the most likely places to uncover them. We are fortunate that among them are various choice edibles.[6–12]

LENTINAN

In the fourteenth century, Chinese physician Wu Rui recorded that shiitake was beneficial in the treatment of various forms of "Malignancy."[13] Likely, he wasn't the only doctor to have found the mushroom sufficiently active against cancer to be noticed. Following their own tests with shiitake against cancers in animals, in a lecture before the Congress of the Hungarian Microbiological Society in 1981, Hungarian scientists Dr. L. Réthy and colleagues announced that the use of fungi in "shamanistic therapy," although principally for treating "tumors," is likely as ancient as humankind. They proclaimed that the recent work in Japan with the shiitake mushroom bore out the folklore as "scientific fact."[14]

Of all the medicinal mushrooms active against tumors, shiitake stands as one of the most intensely studied. The groundbreaking investigation was performed in 1969 by Tetsuro Ikekawa at Purdue University and colleagues at the National Cancer Center Research Institute in Tokyo, Japan's equivalent of the U.S. National Cancer Institute. Shiitake figured among six other edible mushrooms collected in the wilds of Japan, largely at random. They were prepared as water extracts and injected into the stomachs of mice implanted with an intramuscular tumor known as Sarcoma 180. With only one exception, all the mushrooms produced high rates of tumor inhibition (72 to 92 percent),[15] a discovery warmly received by the mushroom-loving Japanese.[16]

TABLE 3

EDIBLE MUSHROOMS WITH ANTITUMOR ACTIVITY[17]

	CURES (%)	TUMOR INHIBITION RATE (%)
Oyster (*Pleurotus ostreatus*)	50	75.3
Shiitake (*Lentinus edodes*)	60	80.7
Enokitake (*Flammulina velutipes*)	30	81.1
Nameko (*Pholiota nameko*)	30	86.5
Matsutake (*Armillaria matsutake*)	55	91.8
Shiitake white powder isolate	66	97.3

Other mushrooms had inhibited the rate at which tumors grew better than shiitake. But when Ikekawa found mice cured in 60 percent of cases in which shiitake was used, more than from any other of the mushroom water extracts, he went on to isolate the active component of shiitake—as yet unidentified polysaccharides in the form of a white powder. When he administered the powder, he found six out of nine mice cured of cancer.[18] The following year an article appeared describing the "highly striking" effects of a particular polysaccharide from shiitake called *lentinan,* so-named after *Lentinus,* the Latin or botanical name for the genus or group of mushrooms shiitake belongs to. For reasons unclear, lentinan showed better antitumor activity in comparatively smaller doses. As little as $\frac{1}{2}$ mg of lentinan per kilogram of body weight had totally regressed Sarcoma 180 tumors in 80 percent of mice, and a 1 mg/kg dose had totally regressed tumors in 100 percent. Signs eventually pointed to an immunologic rather than a chemotherapy-like or cytotoxic action,[19] and this was confirmed in numerous studies that followed.

Since Ikekawa's discovery, dozens upon dozens of scientific articles on lentinan have appeared in journals from countries around the world. The actions of this polysaccharide continue to be a source of inspiration to those in search of safer therapies to combat terminal diseases, and not only in people. On the west coast of Canada, marine biologists recently found lentinan improved the protective effects of vaccines in salmon raised on fish farms.[20] In Japan, lentinan injections alone protected 55 to 75 percent of carp from a lethal bacterial infection.[21] Immune-boosters destined for aquariums? Stay tuned.

Research has shown that lentinan stimulates T-cells, which in turn activate macrophages.[22] Lentinan also stimulates "natural killer" or NK cells,[23] a type of immune cell that plays a critical role in the destruction of tumors and viruses. These cells take on antitumor activity through stimulation by interferon.[24] They kill by way of an enzyme called *perforin*. Perforin makes holes in the outer membrane of enemy cells, causing them to leak and eventually die.[25] The interaction of interferon and NK cells is significant to understanding the body's ability to resist tumor cells and persistent infections by viruses.[26]

LENTINAN IN ACTION

With any drug, no matter how natural, there is always the question of safety. With lentinan, there are no known side effects of any serious nature; those that do occur are mild, of low incidence, and transient.[27–29] Lentinan has produced some outstanding results, in both clinical and laboratory settings. A few are given in the following pages to provide you with a broader view of the actions known.

Combined with some of the more powerful immunobiological drugs available today,[30, 31] lentinan produced significant increases in antitumor effects in animals with tumors caused by carcinogens,[32] and in human endometrial cancer.[33] The combination of lentinan and interleukin 2 (a kind of signaling substance in our immune system that activates immune cells to kill tumors) is so significant that it may well herald "a new avenue of immunotherapy against cancer."[34]

From lentinan alone, gastric carcinoma patients show an increased production of interleukin 1 (IL-1) and tumor necrosis factor (TNF), both substances (produced by monocytes and macrophages) that are known to assist the defense system in the destruction of tumor cells. Lentinan has also elevated the production of interferon and interleukin 2 (IL-2) in cancer patients. Substances known as *cytokines,* IL-2, and interferon in turn stimu-

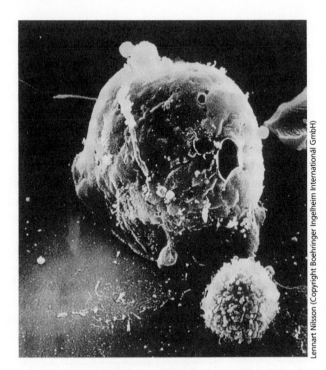

Lennart Nilsson (Copyright Boehringer Ingelheim International GmbH)

Perforated shell of a dead cancer cell with
killer cell resting nearby.

late cells of the immune system. IL-1 stimulates T-cells, partly by inducing the secretion of IL-2. Tumor necrosis factor has a broad spectrum of activity, not the least of which is the activation of immune cells (monocytes and natural killer cells) to directly attack tumor cells. Moreover, tumor necrosis factor has a cell-killing action against tumor cells of its own.[35]

The means by which these mediators stimulate immune cells now appears to be genetically regulated. At least one "major" gene seems to be responsible for the induction of antitumor effects by the immune system from activation by lentinan. Named Ltn-2 after the polysaccharide, that gene offers another important avenue for research in the development of more effective uses of polysaccharides in clinical medicine.[36]

Lentinan has produced some rather unexpected experimental uses, such as the acceleration of bone formation in bone-damaged rats[37] and the therapy and prevention of disseminated intravascular clotting, or sludged blood.[38] And the fact that lentinan is both *immunopotentiating* and *immunorestorative* naturally points to uses beyond cancer. Some have already been found. For example, patients with a drug-resistant strain of tuberculosis that had persisted for over ten years stopped excreting the TB bacterium following treatment with lentinan. Chronic bronchitis in the aged has already shown some good results with lentinan, and other infectious diseases of a chronic nature are undergoing study. Because lentinan induces the production of interferon, it has the added potential of being useful in ongoing battles with viral infections of many kinds.[39]

One U.S. patent proposes the use of lentinan in a cream for cosmetic or medical applications in dermatological disorders. Clinical results from 540 patients found the cream most effective (93 to 100 percent efficient) in treating seborrhea, acne, athlete's foot, male-pattern baldness, and redness of the nose from allergic rhinitis (hay fever). According to the inventors, the cream works by restoring the ionic balance of cell membranes and by exerting osmotic pressure on the inside of the cell membrane.[40]

In Japan, treatment of mice with lentinan prior to radiation provided complete protection from a reduction in white blood cell counts.[41] But in the West we are still in the dark ages; making immunopotentiators available to patients undergoing radiation therapy has yet to be accepted here. There are also documented cases of greatly reduced side effects from radiation and chemotherapy in patients who took herbal immunopotentiators at the same time.[42, 43] Indeed, water extracts of various traditional Chinese herbal formulas have demonstrated radioprotective effects in animals.[44] Protection from radiation exposure is also the subject of ongoing military and space research in the United States, where immunopotentiators are being examined for possible use as radioprotectants in the field. The U.S. Army Medical Research Institute in Frederick, Maryland, determined lentinan to be one of the most active radioprotectors, but application of the findings remains subject to further investigation.[45] The protection of bone marrow cells and their ability to stimulate the production of cytokines appears to be characteristic of immunpotentiators in their ability to provide a radioprotective action.[46, 47]

Patients with recurring breast cancer who received lentinan following surgery had tumor growth regression far greater than what surgery alone could provide.[48] And lentinan may be a preventive in reducing chromosomal damage from anticancer drugs, damage that might otherwise lead to more tumors.[49]

In Japan lentinan is an approved drug for use in the treatment of gastric cancer.[50] Length of life span is significantly longer in patients suffering either recurrent or advanced gastric cancer when they are treated with the chemotherapy agent tegafur[51] or with 5-fluorouracil (with mitomycin C) in combination with lentinan. Without lentinan, neither anticancer agent was as effective.[52] Over 10 percent of those on tegafur combined with lentinan survived over two years, but only 2.9 percent of those on tegafur alone survived the two years,[53] and at the three-year mark there were no survivors on tegafur alone. Also, the tumors were smaller in the combination treatment group.[54] Solid types of gastric tumors are a stubborn sort, with treatments offering a poor rate of survival. One survey revealed that in recurrent gastric cancer the survival rate is only 0.8 percent.[55] But even the 10 percent survival rate from tegafur plus lentinan is poor.

THERAPIES ON THE HORIZON

Lentinan isn't a sure-fire cure for cancer: Japanese Ministry of Health and Welfare drug approval for lentinan was only as an agent to *prolong* survival. A ruling allowing the use of agents to prolong a patient's survival while physicians assess the effectiveness of the chemotherapy applied was only adopted in the United States by the Food and Drug Administration (FDA) in 1985.[56] Thankfully, with that in place we can anticipate life-prolongation agents to increasingly occupy the development of new cancer treatments and perhaps eventually see them used in augmenting old ones.

The focus now and for the future is to find substances with which lentinan can work in concert to enhance recovery from disease. The tactic of applying chemotherapy agents in conjunction with immunostimulants will require considerable care lest the two types of drugs counteract each other. Experiments have shown that in some instances chemotherapy drugs can hamper immune cell destruction of tumor cells, while in other cases such inherently cell-weakening agents can render tumor cells more susceptible to attack by the immune system.[57]

An innovative approach to cancer therapy using immunoactive agents was undertaken by Shigeru Abe at the University of Tokyo in 1982. Dr. Abe explained that alone, immunomodulators have over the long run proven fairly weak against tumors and for this reason have been tested in combination with cytotoxic drugs. Because the immunologic actions of these two kinds of drugs are generally opposed, he felt that such combinations still left something to be desired.[58] What to try next? How about combinations of immunomodulators?

Using another type of immunomodulator known to predominantly effect different kinds of immune cells than those known to be modulated by lentinan, Dr. Abe discovered a greater action from the whole than from the parts. With lentinan plus LPS, a lipopolysaccharide derived from bacteria such as *Escherichia coli*, tumors in mice regressed rapidly, and, in the types of tumors treated, a 77 percent regression in size was much more than either polysaccharide could possibly bring about alone. An "ineffective" amount of LPS had actually *enhanced* the action of lentinan. In fact, either polysaccharide alone had barely caused *any* tumor regressions (in a mammary carcinoma known as MM46 and in Ehrlich's carcinoma).[59] Furthermore, it is well known that LPS, given in *effective* doses, produces too many side effects to qualify for clinical use.

This tactic of combination is reminiscent of a practice inherent to traditional Chinese medicine: herbs with similar immunoactivity are combined to enhance the general resistance or "defenses" of the patient. A significant number of the "defense increasing" or *fu zheng* herbs have demonstrated immunomodulatory effects and have polysaccharides as their most active parts.[60]

Another novel means of potentiating lentinan was found in Japan by one of the country's more prominent surgeons,[61] Dr. Fukumi Morishige, a member of the Linus Pauling Institute[62] and the International Cancer Institute. Following partly successful surgery, a patient was saved from advanced stomach cancer when large doses of vitamin C were given combined with lentinan given intravenously. In Morishige's experience, lentinan has not shown the kind of high rates of antitumor activity in people that occur in animals. He believes this is because animals produce their own vitamin C, and we have to get ours from the environment.[63] This event may lead to further research with vitamin C combined with other kinds of medicinal polysaccharides.

Far away in Chicago, long-term investigations of various natural supplements against terminal cancer now include a shiitake extract. At the Cancer-Care Program at Edgewater Medical Clinic, Director Keith Block, M.D., doesn't think shiitake is a true cure for the disease, but he has found that the mushroom does appear to offer "significant" benefits. Since Dr. Block is an appointed advisor to the Congressional Office of Technology Assessment on Alternative Cancer Treatments,[64] his findings could have a profound effect on future cancer treatments in the United States.

A normal response to disease and disease-causing intruders is a stimulation of the cells that make up that incredibly complex and vast network of cells we simply call the immune system. The collaborative functions of these cells may be likened to a military network, complete with chemical and electronic warfare and an assortment of "agents" feverishly passing intelligence. Because the defensive actions of the system are often insufficient to ward off cancer cells, bacteria, viruses, and pathogenic fungi, the idea of introducing agents to help the body mount a greater immune cell attack was inevitable. Today, immunotherapy provides a supplemental treatment as well as an alternative to the use of strictly cell-toxic drugs, such as those employed in cancer chemotherapy, which are often indiscriminately toxic to normal cells. That is essentially why the interest in immuno-stimulating substances began. Rather than flood the body with massive doses of cytotoxic drugs, the noncytotoxic nature of polysaccharides, for instance, offered a way to destroy unwanted cells without damaging the host.

The isolation and purification of lentinan and much of the clinical research leading to its use as a drug was accomplished through the untiring efforts of Dr. Goro Chihara. At the First International Conference on Mushroom Biology and Mushroom Products in Hong Kong in August 1993, Dr. Chihara criticized the central idea of "killing" cancerous cells with drugs. He stated that we ought instead to be looking for ways to augment defense mechanisms naturally occurring in the body to fight infections and cancerous diseases. To that end he proposes a new term for substances that enhance these mechanisms as "host defense potentiators," or HDPs. Chihara notes that lentinan fulfills this role by potentiating specific immune-activating cells that allow immune cells to respond more effectively against pathogenic cells. He reported that because of this ability, clinical research with lentinan in Japan is currently focusing on preventing cancer from recurring after chemotherapy and surgery. He writes that "the leading principle of the function of lentinan resides in the fact that it can cure patients by restoring their homeostasis, and through enhancement of the intrinsic resistance against diseases." Chihara would like to see the development of other kinds of HDPs that have specific activity in other parts of the system, such as the endocrine and nervous systems, and he acknowledges that in traditional Oriental medicine such agents may already exist and might come to be understood and appreciated by modern biology in the same light.[65]

Dr. Chihara is not alone in this desire, nor the first to present the concept of restoring homeostasis. The question now being asked is which of the diverse cellular mechanisms of the immune system should be modulated in order to restore the natural stability or homeostasis of the system. Some investigators in Japan believe the key lies in the priming of macrophages and related cells and the subsequent production of precursor cells that become mature tumor necrosis factor cells. They propose that many traditional Chinese medicines have performed the task of homeostasis restoration for centuries.[66, 67] Chihara believes that the many different kinds of chemicals responsible for the function of the body, such as neurotransmitters, hormones, and cytokines, which interact with the main cells of the immune system, can only serve in a useful way when the body's *response* to them is completely restored to its "normal state or otherwise enhanced."[68]

FIVE

Cancer Prevention

Reducing the incidence of cancer through diet is a preventive approach many people now readily accept. When the U.S. National Cancer Institute and the American Cancer Society offered the public some dietary guidelines,[1, 2] people began eating more fiber and less fat and selected supplements known to inhibit tumor production.[3, 4] They increased their consumption of tumor-inhibiting vegetables such as broccoli, Brussels sprouts, cauliflower, and cabbage and began taking more vitamins A, C, and E. In all these dietary recommendations shiitake is conspicuously absent, but not for any good reason.[5]

Numerous fruits, vegetables, and some edible seeds (notably sunflower) contain substances that inhibit carcinogen-induced cancers.[6, 7] Cabbage was used in ancient times as a treatment for cancer. Like broccoli, it inhibits cell mutation. In animal experiments, cabbage and broccoli demonstrated remarkable protection against lethal amounts of radiation.[8] As we learned in the last chapter, lentinan from shiitake also has protective effects against carcinogens and radiation damage to the immune system. Yet there are still other cancer preventive substances in this mushroom that everyone ought to know about.

TCA: A NITRITE SCAVENGER

The carcinogenic potential of nitrates and nitrites in our foods is one of those facts of life most would rather not think about. Both get added to bacon and prepared meats to prevent botulism and aflatoxins from forming.[9] Aflatoxins, from the fungus *Aspergillus flavus,* are not only carcinogenic but immunosuppressive, too.[10] The trouble is that nitrites form carcinogenic nitrosamines[11] and nitrate intake and stomach cancer rates are closely correlated.[12] Nitrosamines occur in the stomach by a reaction with amino acids. One often suggested means of protection is to take plenty of vitamin C, about 1 milligram for every milligram of nitrite, or at least 10 mg a day.[13] The vitamin greatly interferes with the formation of nitrosamines in the stomach,[14, 15] although not all of them.[16]

Processed meats are the worst, but they are not the only source of nitrites. Bacteria in the mouth reduce nitrates to nitrites,[17] and some natural compounds in our foods can be converted to carcinogenic mutated forms if treated with nitrites.[18]

For example, the amino acid tyramine (found in cheddar cheese, dried sausage, and many other foods including soy sauce) becomes a carcinogen after mutation induced by treatment with nitrites. As 3-diazothyramine, the mutated amino acid can then induce tumors of the stomach and oral cavity. In Japan, where soy sauce is commonly added to foods, there is a high incidence of stomach cancer and nitrites are highly suspected as the cause. However, other vegetable foods, such as fava beans, have also been found to contain compounds that mutate from exposure to nitrites, and these require further study to determine carcinogenic risk to people ingesting them. In some people nitrites formed in the mouth from nitrates by the reducing action of bacteria are the primary source of nitrite exposure. About 75 percent of nitrite intake in the British diet is from vegetables, particularly lettuce, beet roots, celery, and spinach, and in some vegetables that figure could very well increase with increased use of nitrous fertilizers.[19] A much less publicized source of nitrites is the immune system, where macrophages produce nitrites when they become activated, either by an immunostimulant or as part of their normal attack response to eliminate pathogens.[20–22]

Shiitake can help alleviate the problem posed by nitrites in meats and vegetables, for it contains a substance that scavenges the carcinogenic by-product of nitrites, nitrosamines. That substance is *thioproline,* or TCA.[23] Like vitamin C, it is a naturally occurring antioxidant. It occurs in our bodies, largely in the liver.[24]

An amino acid with a structure similar to penicillin,[25] TCA is a very interesting and valuable compound already developed in Europe as a drug. It isn't difficult to see why.[26] TCA has shown liver-protectant effects against various commonly consumed chemicals (acetominophen, tetracycline, and ethanol),[27] and it suppressed (by 78 percent) the formation of cancer cells in animals exposed to carcinogenic nitrite compounds in the diet.[28] In diluted amounts (1 part to 500), TCA is patented in Japan for use in controlling fungal infection in rice plants.[29] In old animals, TCA significantly stimulated enzymatic activities in the liver toward levels found in young animals.[30] In high doses (100 to 400 mg/day) in tablet form, TCA has been used in the treatment of liver diseases and as a drug to counteract aging.[31] A similar compound made in the United States and called OTC or Procysteine is the subject of clinical research in AIDS patients, where it may be useful for increasing both the resistance to oxidation of normal cells by unpaired electrons (free radicals) that run rampant in the body with this disease, and the responsiveness of T-cells.[32]

The TCA in shiitake traps nitrites in the body, allowing them to be removed in the urine. Otherwise, they will form carcinogenic compounds, largely in the stomach. But there's a trick to taking advantage of this: the mushroom must be dried but not powdered, and then cooked. Powdering the mushroom destroys enzymes needed to form TCA.[33]

If you were to analyze fresh shiitake for TCA, you wouldn't find any, but you don't need to be an alchemist to produce it. TCA doesn't reach detectable limits until the mushroom gets boiled for at least five to eight minutes. The amount in dried shiitake isn't always detectable either, but after boiling, it goes up dramatically. Even soaking the dried mushroom for half an hour improves the TCA level. Using 5 grams shiitake per 50 ml of water, the quantity of TCA reaches 7 µg per gram.[34]

Now, a wonderful thing happens when the right foods are combined with the mushroom in cooking: the level of TCA goes up even higher. The secret is to cook the mushroom with foods rich in the amino acid cysteine. The National Cancer Center Research Institute (NCCRI) in Tokyo learned that if dried shiitake (100 grams, or about 30 mushrooms) were cooked with chicken liver (100 grams), a rich source of cysteine, the amount of

TCA produced from the mushroom would reach about 10 mg. That increase represents a jump of over fourteen times the TCA found in the soaked mushroom, and that much TCA would increase the Japanese average twelve-hour urinary excretion of nitrite by over 300 percent! The NCCRI concluded that the "TCA generated from edible amounts of [shiitake] mushroom can actually contribute to the trapping of nitrite in the human body." In fact, other than frozen cod, no food in the Japanese diet contains so much TCA.[35]

VITAMIN D

Scientists who study the incidence of disease have cited the possibility of too little vitamin D in our diets as a primary factor in higher incidences of breast cancer and, it seems, of colon cancer.[36–40] Vitamin D has shown antitumor activity in rats with mammary tumors[41] and inhibited the formation of colon tumors in rats in which tumor formation was promoted by giving them a diet high in fat. Curiously, tumor inhibition was not found in rats on a low-fat diet supplemented with vitamin D.[42]

Researchers at the University of California at San Diego noticed that in areas with the least sunlight—our main source of vitamin D—or even where sunlight is more blocked because of air pollution, the incidence of these cancers is higher. The death rate from breast cancer in New York, for example, is over 1.5 times the rate in Hawaii and Phoenix, Arizona.[43] The D-factor also appears elsewhere in the world. From 1969 to 1971, rates of breast cancer in fifteen republics of the former Soviet Union were highest in those that had the smallest amounts of sunlight. And just as those republics that received intermediate amounts of sunlight had correspondingly intermediate rates of breast cancer, those receiving the most sunlight had the least incidence.[44] A larger study, with 25,620 people over eight years in the United States, found that those who developed colon cancer had significantly lower serum levels of vitamin D during the same period.[45] In examining rates of breast cancer for eighty-seven regions of the United States, vitamin D appears to be a much stronger factor than fat intake. Even red meat consumption, which is fairly uniform throughout the country, doesn't correlate with the difference in regional incidence.[46]

In the northern zones, where sunlight is at lower levels, Japan remains the exception; there, the lower incidence in both kinds of cancer is attributed to higher consumption of vitamin D–rich fish oil.[47] In a Chicago population studied for nineteen years, those who had a minimum daily intake of 150 IU of the vitamin had half the colon cancer rate as those who took less. Just why hasn't been worked out, but the U.S. National Institutes of Health is now investigating the matter.[48]

Actions on the immune system will be a major area of focus because not only are there places (receptors) specifically designed by nature for vitamin D to directly interact on the surface of lymphocytes,[49] but vitamin D_3 (a hormone otherwise known as calcitriol, a metabolite of the vitamin primarily produced by skin exposure to sunlight) has been found to enhance natural killer cell activity in patients who have depressed levels of NK cell action.[50] Studies have also shown that vitamin D_3 is a potent NK cell activity stimulant and that it seems to enhance these cells by augmenting macrophages to release an NK cell stimulating factor.[51] A single large oral dose (600,000 IU) of vitamin D_3 given to patients with low levels of T-cells (cases of osteoporosis and of bone fractures) restored T-cell counts to normal levels, but the same dose did not increase T-cell numbers in healthy people.[52]

A single shiitake mushroom may contain 56 IU of vitamin D or more.[53] In one analysis,[54] the amount of vitamin D in only 2 grams of sunlight-irradiated shiitake was 360 IU, which is only 40 IU short of the U.S. recommended daily allowance and more than double what the subjects in Chicago with noticeably less colon cancer were taking.[55]

FOOD FOR THE IMMUNE SYSTEM

In 1974 Kisaku Mori reported that he had found various instances of the shiitake mushroom being "helpful" against leukemia[56] and stomach cancer.[57] About ten years later, shiitake gained the attention of an American physician as the result of a similar occurrence. A patient diagnosed with a malignancy had unexpectedly started to improve at the same time a shiitake extract entered the diet.[58] An extract of the mycelium has its share of cases, too. According to a U.S. patent for the extract, in 1977 physicians in Japan documented two patients who had complete cures of cancer (pancreatic and esophageal) from taking a mere 6 grams of the extract (orally) each day before breakfast. The extract was administered on humanitarian grounds—a last ditch effort to provide the patients with *something*—even though they were not expected to survive. The patient with cancer of the esophagus had refused conventional treatments, and the patient with malignant, migrating pancreatic cancer had two masses of tumor, each the size of a fist.[59] Intriguing as they are, however, anecdotal accounts of a mushroom affecting cancer in people are not going to be taken very seriously unless they can be backed up with controlled studies.

Unequivocal proof of antitumor activity from eating the mushroom was finally established in 1986. The investigation was conducted by the son of Kisaku Mori, Kanichi Mori of the Mushroom Research Institute of Japan, in conjunction with Professor Hiroaki Nanba of the Kobe Women's College of Pharmacy. They revealed their unprecedented results at an international symposium on edible mushrooms held at Pennsylvania State University. Here's what they found:

Without the mushroom as part of the diet, Sarcoma 180 tumors in mice grew without restraint. But with 10 percent of their feed consisting of shiitake powder, tumor growth was inhibited by almost 40 percent. With a diet of 30 percent shiitake powder, the results were more impressive. The researchers found over 58 percent fewer tumor cells in one group, and 66.7 and 77.9 percent fewer in other groups on the same amount of shiitake.[60]

It was evident that tumor suppression increased the longer the mice were given shiitake. But why? Efforts were made to determine whether something apart from the obvious might be involved. A whole-shiitake powder supplement in the diet resulted in 66.7 percent fewer tumors, but with the polysaccharides removed the rate dropped to only 38.9 percent. Besides polysaccharides, shiitake contains lipids, or fat. When the researchers used defatted shiitake in the feed, the rate of tumor growth dropped again, by about 10 percent. Little tumor inhibition was found when the normal feed was supplemented with the shiitake fat alone (only 24.7 percent); however, it was enough to conclude that tumor suppression from ingesting shiitake was the result of *both* lipids and polysaccharides.[61]

Meticulous testing revealed that the immune system was being significantly activated, which was the only reasonable explanation for the poor growth in tumors.[62] Upon further testing, the immune cells responsible were identified as macrophages, natural killer cells, and T-cells.[63, 64]

The macrophage is a type of white blood cell known as a phagocyte, a name taken from the Greek *phago,* meaning to eat, and *cyt,* meaning cell. Much like the video game character "Pac Man," they go around eating and disposing of foreign invaders such as microorganisms, dust particles in the lungs, pathogenic fungi, contaminants from smoke, and just about anything else they are able to determine might be a burden to the health of the body. These dragons of the immune system occur in large numbers where there is chronic inflammation. They flock to wound sites or lesions where bacteria and other foreign invaders can enter to cause infections. These cells gobble up the intruders until they finally eat themselves— sacrificing themselves for the well-being of the body.

Besides the bloodstream, macrophages have as their main sites in the body a large territory that includes the spleen, bone marrow, lymph nodes, air sacs in the lungs (pulmonary alveoli), peritoneum (the membrane lining the abdominal wall), liver, connective tissue, and central nervous system. In keeping infections at bay and—if sufficiently stimulated—killing cancer cells, the macrophage is of prime importance. Unless they are activated, how-ever, macrophages lie dormant in the body.

Researchers Mori and Nanba found that the tumor-cell–destroying ac-tion of macrophages appeared after the mice had eaten shiitake for twelve days. At that point tumorcidal activity reached 1.8 times normal, enough also to inhibit a type of breast cancer (MM46 carcinoma) at a rate of close to 79 percent.[65] Because natural killer cells act on the very front lines of the immune system to combat virus-infected and tumor cells, the researchers suspected NK cell activation was involved in the breast cancer inhibition. Mice with the breast cancer were divided into two groups; one group was fed shiitake for one week, and the other was given normal feed. After a week, their levels of natural killer cell activation were measured. By about the eighth day, the level of activity had risen to almost twice normal and then dropped back to normal. By day 21, the NK cell activity in tumor-bearing mice on ordinary feed fell all the way to 21 percent of normal, but

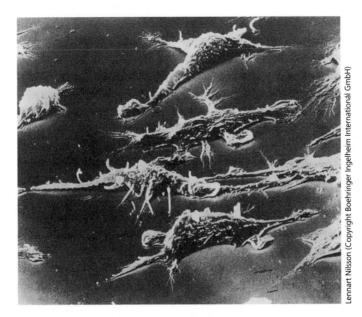

Lennart Nilsson (Copyright Boehringer Ingelheim International GmbH)

Dragon-like macrophages at rest.

the level of NK cell activity of those on shiitake feed fell more slowly and then only as far as 71 percent of normal.[66]

Next, the researchers examined for T-cell activity. Mice with tumor cells fed on shiitake feed for two weeks and a day. Now in addition to macrophage and NK cell activation, the activity of T-cells had increased 1.4 times. The researchers concluded that ingestion of shiitake fruit-bodies seems to parallel the kind of immune cell activation produced by injections of lentinan.[67]

Along with their ally the macrophage, T-cells gang up to fight the body's greatest battles. They are known as T-cells because they undergo maturation in the thymus. T-cells take "intelligence" garnered by the macrophage from undesirable cells, recognize the nature of these cells through the information transmitted, and then alert a rapid-attack kind of T-cell called killer T-cells. These troops multiply quickly and in vast numbers, taking the intelligence passed to identify and destroy the exact kind of undesirables spotted by the macrophage. Little wonder the immune system came to be known as our second brain.

The bit of intelligence is something called *antigen*. Antigens are found on the surface of viruses, tumor cells, microorganisms, and a myriad of potential disease-causing agents. In short, T-cells react to antigen by producing substances (cytokines such as interleukin 2) that stimulate attacks and "intelligence-relay" by an assortment of other immune cells, including macrophages. Once activated by T-cells, the macrophage goes into high gear, developing a wide spectrum of activity against tumor cells.

MEDICINAL MYCELIUM

The mycelium offers a further source of cancer preventive food. In a bagasse-and-rice-bran medium used to grow shiitake, another team of researchers discovered several anticarcinogenic substances. The source of the anticarcinogens was an extract of the mycelium dubbed *Lentinus edodes* mycelial extract, or LEM for short. LEM is a water-soluble extract of the mycelium made before the fruit-bodies have had a chance to form. LEM-treated rats feeding on a carcinogen as part of their food showed as much as 50 percent less proliferation of cancer.[68] Later, colon tumors resulting from a carcinogen were treated with the extract, and the number of tumors diminished.[69]

One of the antitumor factors in the mycelium of shiitake is the polysaccharide *emitanin* (37.5 mg per gram of mycelium).[70] Emitanin was patented in Japan for use against cancer in 1977. In animals, this polysaccharide (10 mg/kg of body weight) caused good rates of tumor inhibition, which ranged from 63 to 82 percent.[71]

There are also reports of polysaccharides from the mycelium that exhibit activity against liver cancer resulting from a carcinogen.[72] One of those, a water-soluble, peptide-containing polysaccharide known as KS-2, holds potent antitumor activity and is active by the oral route. Not many polysaccharide compounds are. KS-2 caused interferon production in cancer patients and suppressed tumor growth in mice. With an oral dose of as little as 1 mg/kg, KS-2 had a very strong inhibitory effect against the Sarcoma 180 tumor; all the mice survived. Mice with a much more difficult to survive cancer (Ehrlich ascitic tumors) required a higher oral dose of KS-2 (140 mg/kg), but even after fifty days—twenty days longer than most antitumor studies wait for results—70 percent had survived. Afterward, their macrophages were examined. As proof of immunostimulation, when placed among tumor cells, the macrophages started to kill the abnormal cells.[73]

Largely made up of the simple sugar mannose, KS-2 is a polysaccharide bound to proteins and peptides and consists of a wide range of amino acids. KS-2 suppresses tumor growth when taken orally in doses of 1 to 140 mg/kg, yet it has an extremely low level of toxicity: oral doses of more than 12,500 mg per kilogram of body weight were required before problems appeared in mice.[74] Another form, called KS-2-B, has fewer amino acids and appears slightly more active. The KS stands for Kirin-Seagram, the companies that arranged for the research and patented the compound.[75] Kirin is famous for its beer, and Seagram makes whiskey. Other distilleries could take a lesson from them: it was the waste grain used in whiskey production on which they grew shiitake mycelium to obtain KS-2.

PROOF IN PEOPLE

Even after all these proofs in animals, there was still no research on immunological effects in people consuming shiitake, the deciding frontier. This was largely because of the expense. We are fortunate indeed to have even one study. It proved that eating shiitake daily really does give the immune system a boost.

A clinical investigation was quietly conducted by a private biomedical company in the United States over a period of four years.[76] In total, 116 people were examined, 105 of whom served as control subjects so there could be no doubt of the results, whatever might be found. When normal people ingested the powdered fruit-body daily, 1 teaspoonful (1,500 mg) a day,[77] their levels of helper T-cells showed a "statistically significant increase" compared to two groups of control subjects not taking the mushroom.[78] Depending on the size of the mushrooms, a gram and a half (1,500 mg) of dried shiitake is only about four mushrooms. A handful a day isn't a lot to take. And in the more convenient extract form of shiitake fruit-body, the equivalent of 1,500 mg of dried mushroom might be obtained from 150 mg.

Also called CD4+T-lymphocytes, helper T-cells were so named because they literally help other immune cells to attack foreign cells. Other kinds of T-cells primarily kill foreign cells, and when there is too much activation, to keep the immune system in balance some suppress immune cell activity. As with the mice in Japan with shiitake in their feed, higher helper T-cell counts occurred in patients who had longer ingested the mushroom. In two patients, helper T-cell counts dropped sharply after only two weeks off the mushroom,[79] telling us only that in some people blood counts will return to normal more rapidly than in others.

Results with lentinan are similar but not exactly the same. Daily oral doses in rats most significantly elevated helper T-cell counts; however, at the eighth week they developed tolerance to lentinan,[80, 81] which means that their systems no longer responded to it. Similar findings with other immunomodulators[82, 83] have led some to suggest intermittent or *pulsed* dosing, such as half the dose for a month following two months of the full dose, or a break from the agent for a month.[84] Others propose this in addition to taking an agent every other day instead of daily.

SIX

Warring With Viruses

Shiitake joined in the war on AIDS in 1983, when lentinan was successful in the treatment of a patient with HIV in Japan[1, 2]—so successful that the patient no longer had the disease. HIV-positive readings gradually disappeared in direct parallel with an array of abnormalities until all returned to normal.[3, 4] Few people outside of AIDS researchers seem to know about the case, but it isn't as if the treatment has been kept secret. The entire world was told when the results were presented in 1985 at the Third International Conference on Immunopharmacology in Florence, Italy.

The patient, a woman of fifty-seven, showed positive to HIV and to the T-cell leukemia virus, HTLV-I. She had enlarged lymphatic glands and lower than normal helper T-cells (15.9 percent) and NK cell activity (36 percent).[5] The leukemia virus (HTLV-1) in a patient positive for HIV causes AIDS to develop much faster, a fact that only emerged five years later. This was the first definite viral cofactor identified in the development of AIDS.[6]

Now afflicting people from the South American Andes to the islands of Japan and the streets of New York and Los Angeles, HTLV-I has existed almost throughout the world for thousands of years and can be passed in the same ways as the AIDS virus.[7, 8] Because the virus mutates, some scientists warn of a possible HTLV-I epidemic, right on the heels of AIDS.[9] Like HIV, which belongs to the same family of viruses, in parts of the world where sexual transmission rates are higher from unprotected sex with multiple partners, HTLV-I appears to have greater virulence.[10] And it is more than a cofactor in AIDS. Apart from leukemia, the virus causes an inflammatory disorder of the eyes (uveitis),[11] cancer of the lymph nodes (lymphoma),[12, 13] and something called TSP (tropical spastic paraparesis),[14] a paralyzing, degenerative neurological disease that resembles chronic multiple sclerosis. But let's get back to the fortunate patient in Japan.

Following a breast cancer operation over a year earlier, at which time radiation had been applied as a follow-up treatment, she was admitted for lentinan therapy to correct "progressive weakness." How the HIV was contracted isn't known for certain. One possibility, put forward by her physicians, was the blood transfusion she received during the operation for breast cancer.[15]

After regular injections of lentinan (1 mg intravenously by drip infusion two times a week) for five months, readings for the viruses were restored to negative. The helper T-cell population noticeably improved (to 23 percent), and NK cell activity rose dramatically (from 36 to 80.8 percent).[16] Three years after the treatment, the patient was still healthy,[17] without requiring further use of the drug.[18] Her case made history in the annals of medicine, representing the first reported occurrence of HIV in Japan.[19]

Three years later, lentinan was approved by the government for national investigative treatment of the syndrome in Japan.[20] The first clinical trial results were from hemophiliacs accidently infected with HIV. In less than twelve weeks, some lymphocytic cells were restored almost to normal. This resulted in open trials of lentinan for HIV in sixteen medical universities and hospitals throughout Japan.[21]

Literally thousands of articles on AIDS research appear every month, and even doctors who treat AIDS can't keep up. But today a growing number of healthcare professionals know lentinan holds promise,[22] especially in stimulating[23] and restoring[24] the helper T-cell. Lentinan ranks as the first immuno-drug on record to increase the cell-killing ability of T-cells by restoring function of the helper T-cell.[25, 26] In Japan, two out of four HIV-positive hemophiliacs maintained the increase in their helper T-cells from lentinan.[27] As a result, clinical trials of lentinan in AIDS were begun in the United States in 1989. In a pilot study, 30 percent of the patients showed an increasing level of helper T-cells.[28–30]

The emphasis on increasing helper T-cell counts is now becoming only secondarily indicative of therapeutic gains from a treatment but will continue to be watched as one sign of improvement. This is because of evidence that the pool of T-cells in AIDS patients can be greatly depleted by the attack of HIV on the macrophage and dendritic cells, macrophage-like cells largely found in the lymph nodes and skin. These cells present antigen to the immune system, which, as a result, normally becomes stimulated and remembers to send the message to produce T-cells to attack the viruses and other foreign cells. A defect in this antigen-presenting function could muzzle immune system memory enough to keep T-cell production down. In AIDS, this theory would partly explain why although only a small number of T-cells are infected with HIV, the disease progresses.[31, 32]

In the context of developing treatments for AIDS, it is interesting to note that unlike T-cells, the macrophage can live on even though infected with HIV. When T-cells are stimulated, they proliferate and the infection process goes into a higher gear and then kills them. But not so for the macrophage. When HIV-infected macrophages were subjected to immuno-stimulants, HIV production decreased. Curiously, the cell-killing actions one would normally expect to be responsible for virus destruction by the macrophage—such as phagocytosis and the production of free radical electrons, which the macrophage deploys to zap intruders—couldn't account for the down-regulation of HIV production. At the time of this writing, it appears that the macrophage harbors some unknown mechanisms that can substantially hamper the proliferation of HIV.[33] This finding may provide further reason for scientists to study the clinical application of lentinan in the various stages of AIDS progression, for the polysaccharide is a potentiator of both T-cells and macrophages.

Much better results are expected from combining lentinan with antiviral drugs. Laboratory results showed that by itself, lentinan has no HIV-infection–blocking action in the test tube. One would expect this from an immunomodulator, since they act by way of the immune system. But applied at the same time as azidothymidine (AZT), the most widely prescribed antiviral drug for AIDS, lentinan augmented the antiviral. In fact, neither AZT nor lentinan was anywhere near as effective as when they were combined.[34] AZT plus lentinan was five to twenty-four times more effective at inhibiting HIV than AZT alone.[35]

This strategy is now being used in long-term, carefully controlled studies at several hospitals in the United States. These trials are being sponsored by Bristol-Meyers Squibb, Lentico-Chemico of New Jersey, and lentinan's manufacturer, Ajinomoto of Japan. Patients are given the polysaccharide by itself or in combination with a drug called ddl or Videx.[36] Like AZT, this agent inhibits an enzyme system that HIV uses to replicate itself;[37] however, ddl doesn't appear to be as toxic as AZT.[38, 39] To date, few immune-enhancing drugs have been tested in AIDS. They often meet with prejudice in the United States, regardless of mounting evidence of their benefits in Europe and Japan. But then, in medicine, prejudice often precedes inquiry.[40]

HIV MEETS THE MYCELIUM

The mycelial extract was once largely unknown in the United States to all but AIDS patients. Because it poses no problems of toxicity, people in many parts of the world today are asking how it might benefit them.

The invention of the extract was completely unintentional. It all started some twenty years ago when an electrical engineer in Japan, Chiyokichi Iizuka, was trying to sell freezers to the mushroom industry. He was looking for a way to preserve exotic mushrooms until the expensive season when supply is limited and prices soar. That led him to find a way of growing shiitake artificially, without the use of logs, the slow traditional method. Because trees were becoming scarce and the old method takes years, he had plenty of incentive. Then he toyed with the idea of extracting shiitake to produce a flavoring agent, and with that came a liquid culture method. But he never did go into the flavoring business. People were telling him that their ailments improved when they drank the mushroom liquid, so he brought out a beverage form of the mycelium,[41-44] which is enjoyed in Japan to this day.

But Iizuka still managed to cultivate the mushroom. Instead of logs or sawdust, he decided on using rice bran and leftover sugar cane, or bagasse, an inexpensive growing medium rich in natural sugars. He knew that in Japan a drink prepared from boiled bagasse had, coincidentally,

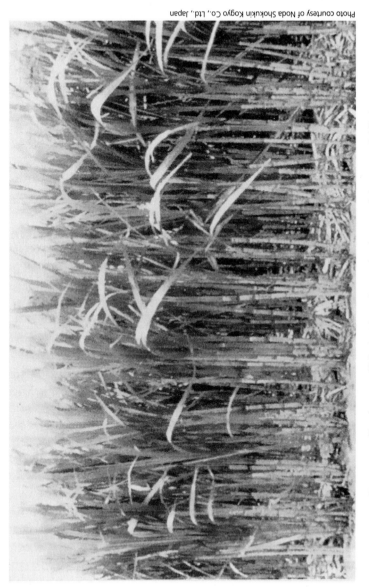

Sugar cane (Saccharum officinale L.) used to make the mycelial extract of shiitake.

been an old folk remedy for cancer. After harvesting the mushrooms, he had to dispose of the leftover mycelium. He wondered, Could it be used as a fertilizer? To find out, he offered it to a nearby farmer, who suggested he spread it around his tobacco crop. The tobacco was afflicted with a viral infection (tobacco mosaic virus) that also affects tomatoes and green peppers. The plants weren't going to make it anyway, and the farmer didn't want to take a chance with something untried on his good plants. To everyone's amazement, the crop healed and was harvested. Iizuka learned that even after five dilutions, the extract continued to exhibit revitalizing effects. Later, rice and vegetable crops were treated with the extract, and their yields increased. Cancer and viral disease research became a logical progression.[45]

The mycelial extract, often referred to as LEM, is still produced using bagasse shavings and rice bran in a liquid shiitake culture. It sits for months digesting in its own enzymes. This process breaks down the cell walls of the mycelium, liberating the active constituents within. The water is then removed, and the extract is freeze-dried to produce a convenient granular powder.[46]

In Kyoto, at the First Conference of AIDS Researchers, held in December 1987, Dr. Naoki Yamamoto of Yamaguchi University School of Medicine disclosed that LEM had "very effectively" interfered with HIV in a series of laboratory tests. Dr. T. S. Tochikura, a foremost expert on medical fungi who had been in charge of the research, concluded that the results with LEM suggest that the extract may "inhibit virus replication during a very early stage of the replication cycle" of HIV. LEM inhibited the virus from spreading either cell to cell or in a cell-free manner, the two main ways HIV travels in its cycle of infection and replication.[47] He also found the mycelial extract to be less toxic and more effective than AZT.[48] In the same year, Harumi Suzuki at the University of Tokyo reported that parts of LEM had activated macrophages and had caused bone marrow cells to proliferate.[49] Since the bone marrow is where immune cells literally form themselves,[50] his finding is one of great significance.

Of these parts of LEM that had activated macrophages, something called EP3 proved highly active against HIV in the laboratory.[51, 52] Not only was the enzyme system that HIV uses to make copies of itself in the body inhibited (by 90 percent), but EP3 also "completely inhibited" the cell-damaging effect of HIV to highly sensitive T-cells. Naturally, the researchers wondered whether EP3 would affect other viruses, and it did. It provided complete inhibition of cell-damaging effects from herpes simplex (types I and II), as well as from a virus that causes encephalitis in horses (Western equine encephalitis virus). It also provided partial inhibition of mumps virus, measles virus, and polio virus.[53]

EP3 turned out to be both *immunostimulating* and *antiviral*. Suzuki's team expected to find the main immuno-active part of LEM to be a polysaccharide, but instead they discovered a lignin, and an antiviral one at that.[54] EP3 is made up of several lignins, which originate not in the mushroom mycelium but in the spent sugar cane used to grow the mycelium.[55] Tests to find which organs in the body these water-soluble lignins travel to when taken orally revealed that they reach maximum absorption in six hours, with the largest quantities found in the liver, lymph nodes, kidney cortex, and vertebra. EP3 stayed in the kidney cortex, vertebra, and lymph nodes longer than in the liver.[56]

Polysaccharides and lignins are the main components of dietary fiber. Lignins make up as much as 30 percent of the woody cells of trees, and along with cellulose (a polysaccharide) they form the cell walls of wood. Lignins are complex aromatic substances occurring in woody plants throughout the world. They are some of the toughest natural substances on the planet and are usually not soluble in water.

As early as 1968, an antitumor lignin was isolated in Japan from bamboo grass (*Sasa kurilensis*).[57] But as a class of compounds lignins have until very recently been largely neglected in medical research. Today, the purified antiviral and immunoactive parts of LEM are undergoing further tests to develop useful nontoxic agents to combat viral diseases.[58, 59] A protein-bound polysaccharide (glycoprotein) showed antiviral activity,[60] but the most active of LEM derivatives is a water soluble lignin naturally attached to proteins and polysaccharides.[61]

Based upon the pronounced action of the lignin against HIV, a study was conducted in HIV-positive hemophiliacs. The daily dose of LEM was

9 grams. In two patients with full-blown AIDS, yeast infection (candidiasis) was relieved, "clinical symptoms" improved, and lymphocyte activity was "markedly enhanced."[62]

Akira Shirahata, who headed up the study, concluded that LEM, being "remarkably efficient" at increasing the activity of patients' lymphocytes and having improved the symptoms of both AIDS patients, is worthy of being applied "to try to prevent development of AIDS and to treat the disease."[63]

According to these results, LEM may be useful for people with the same yeast infection but who don't have AIDS. As added proof, in mice first given cortisone as an immunosuppressant, yeast infection caused by the pathogenic fungus *Candida albicans* caused their level of vitality to drop. When LEM was given following two weeks of the infection, 100 percent of their vitality was restored.[64]

Largely because of the successes reported in Japan, people with AIDS and others who are positive for HIV but haven't yet shown major symptoms are taking about 2 grams of LEM a day until symptoms abate without relapse (guesstimated at six months to a year), then allowing a maintenance dose of 650 mg a day.[65] Tests for toxicity found LEM to be virtually "as safe as a general food."[66]

Three cases, fairly representative of the results in Japan, were found in a small trial of the extract in the United States. The trial was conducted by Dr. Kevin Jones of Emperor's College of Traditional Oriental Medicine in Santa Monica, California. No side effects were found in any of the cases.[67, 68]

In Jones's first case, an AIDS patient with Kaposi's sarcoma tumors showed a reading of 822 helper T-cells before receiving LEM. After LEM (9 grams a day taken orally for 90 days), the helper T-cell count rose to 1,050. As noted earlier, a rise in helper T-cell counts is now considered a general indication of improvement. The normal count is around 400 to 1,400 in men and 400 to 1,800 in women. Major AIDS symptoms usually occur at around 200. But a more telling indicator of AIDS progression is Kaposi's sarcoma, which is a definite sign of full-blown AIDS. This patient unfortunately developed complications from pneumonia and could not be saved despite the improvement.[69]

The second AIDS patient showed a helper T-cell count of 1,250 cells, along with fever and fatigue. After two months on LEM (6 grams a day), the count was 2,542, and the fever and fatigue were relieved. In the third case of an AIDS carrier (HIV-positive but without symptoms), following 6 grams a day for two months antigen for the virus could not be found: the patient had become HIV-negative.[70]

Dr. Jones now gives HIV-positive patients a basic experimental protocol consisting of acupuncture (two or three times a week), a vitamin C complex (oral, 5 to 20 grams a day), and the mycelial extract, 18 grams a day.[71]

People with HIV who have outlived the average time of death after HIV infection of about five years, commonly known as long-term AIDS survivors, are now, finally, the subject of ongoing studies by the U.S. National Institutes of Health. Because some of these subjects have a history of taking unconventional antiviral substances and immunopotentiators such as acemannan, a polysaccharide derived from aloe vera and similar in some ways to lentinan, in 1993 NIH scientists began planning clinical trials using the same unconventional compounds.[72]

Since the discovery that HIV-positive patients without symptoms harbor HIV in their macrophages[73] and lymphoid tissues (lymph nodes, spleen, tonsils, and adenoids)—until the immune system becomes so impaired that it spills out[74-76]—AIDS scientists are saying that instead of waiting for T-cell counts to drop, patients may soon be treated straightaway. So it seems the tactic of applying life-prolongation agents—resisted for so long in the United States—may finally catch on. That opens the possibility of a patient never having symptoms if treated early enough.

Now the search is on for drugs that won't destroy the body even when taken for many years, certainly for decades and perhaps a lifetime.[77] Such drugs would need to be practically as safe as a food, antiviral, and immunopotentiating. Any treatment will very likely involve several agents. Shiitake and its various nontoxic by-products will undoubtedly become strong candidates for study, as will many other natural products already researched in AIDS but so far neglected by mainstream Western medicine.

HEPATITIS AND HERPES

In the United States, over 500,000 people a year are infected with hepatitis, and 16,000 die, mostly from the hepatitis B virus.[78, 79] One in twenty Americans has been exposed, and it is now known that exposure is largely (41 percent) through heterosexual activity. The fact that for 26 percent the means of exposure remains to be known tells us that we have a lot to learn about this virus before we can get it under control.[80]

According to the Centers for Disease Control and Prevention (CDCP), about 1.25 million Americans are now carriers of hepatitis B.[81] The CDCP is sufficiently concerned to recommend routine vaccination for all babies.[82] Worldwide, over one million die every year, and at least 300 million are infected, making hepatitis the world's most prevalent disease.[83] About 30 percent of infected individuals become *chronic active hepatitis* patients, in which the disease can graduate to liver cancer, cirrhosis, and liver failure. Alpha-interferon injections (approved in 1992) are only 40 percent effective at putting the disease into remission.[84] Medicinal plants are a relatively new arena in the search for substances that may contribute to the regression of the disease.[85]

The mycelial extract may be a real boon in the treatment of viral hepatitis.[86] Trials of LEM at sixteen clinics in Japan found that it causes protective antibodies to form in patients with chronic type hepatitis B. In one pilot study in 40 patients on LEM for four months (6 grams orally per day), the patients with chronic active hepatitis showed a 36.8 percent rate of seroconversion, meaning that in those cases the virus changed to an inactive type.[87] In other studies, in as little as three months (5 grams orally per day), LEM had completely cured patients with severe epidemic forms of the disease, "indicating an astonishingly high therapeutic effect." This followed positive results with the extract in suppressing the formation of liver cancer as well as the spread of existing liver cancer cells in animals.[88] While LEM enhances antibody response,[89] it may also act as a liver cell protectant against autoimmune damage, in which the immune system attacks normal cells, mistaking their diseased forms for invading cells. Indeed, autoimmune damage is now a suggested means of liver cell damage in hepatitis B.[90]

Another rapidly spreading virus, herpes, may also contribute to AIDS progression,[91] and LEM holds compounds that inhibit the infectious actions of that virus, too. One of the components responsible is *zeatin,* a growth-stimulating substance of plants. Zeatin was named after *Zea mays,* or sweet corn, the plant from which it was originally isolated.[92]

The herpes-preventive action of zeatin produced better, even "excellent" results when the polysaccharide component of LEM was combined with it. According to researchers in Japan, who after repeated tests went on to patent the application, without the mixture of polysaccharides and zeatin only 10 percent of mice survived. But if the combination was administered, even two days after a lethal dose of herpes, 75 percent survived. If the mixture was given two days before infection, 90 percent survived.[93] Those results are extremely good for any substance tested against herpes, and they are especially high for something nontoxic.

The whole antiherpes part or fraction of LEM, dubbed JLS-18 by its discoverers, is rich in water-soluble lignin (65 to 75 percent), polysaccharides (15 to 30 percent), and peptides (10 to 20 percent). It has been shown that this fraction can be effectively applied against herpes topically, or when taken orally. Not only does this part of LEM inhibit the ability of herpes to replicate and thereby multiply in the body, it also inhibits the recurrence of outbreaks in a previously infected host. Taken orally by mice infected with herpes simplex, 500 µg of the fraction a day for five days caused all the mice to produce negative readings for the virus in their blood three weeks later. The inventors add that owing to its high stability, JLS-18 could be made up into a wide variety of preparations, including tablets, powders, granules, "lemonades," creams, and ointments, and that to treat outbreaks topical preparations need contain only 0.01 to 1 percent of the substance.[94]

At the Department of Internal Medicine of Chigasaki Municipal Hospital in Japan, Dr. Kijuro Nomura noted favorable responses to the mycelial extract in patients with nasal allergies, skin allergies, allergies in general, asthma, and viral hepatitis. In view of his observations, a pilot study of LEM in similar cases was conducted by Emperor's College. There were ten patients with herpes of the genitals, four allergy patients, and one with eczema. One herpes patient also had AIDS. Other than a single case of diarrhea, the treatment was free of side effects.[95] The clinical report concluded as follows:

> One patient experienced a reaction before improvement started. This may seem, if it is not understood, to be a worsening of the condition. However, after a few days improvements were monitored. In cases of Herpes simplex II most of the patients suffered a great deal from severe pain. Some of these patients improved rapidly after beginning treatment.[96]

Following three months of treatment (9 g of LEM per day), the patient with eczema and every allergy patient had improved. Of the herpes patients, 30 percent improved considerably, 30 percent improved moderately, and 10 percent stabilized their disease.[97] The rest, while not showing visible signs of improvement, experienced "no aggravation" of their disease.[98] A press release on this study provides further hope that this simple food may become an invaluable aid to the virally infected:

> Significant in the AIDS patient was that the T-cell count increased with special note that the T-helper population increased. This indicates a trend reversal of the syndrome and is especially important because as these vital cells decrease, the AIDS patients become more susceptible to other viruses and opportunistic infections.
>
> One herpes patient, who requested to be unidentified, noted that his symptoms "disappeared," and called the substance "fantastic." The AIDS patient, also requesting anonymity, told his doctor that he was feeling more energy and overall improved.[99]

An inherent lack of toxicity should be reason enough for the continued study of shiitake products, which may bring options to millions afflicted with this virus alone. In the United States, at least 40 million people are now infected with genital herpes, and 500,000 more cases appear each year. Orthodox physicians offer nothing to cure what is indisputably the most prevalent venereal disease in our society.[100, 101]

SEVEN

Chronic Fatigue Syndrome

At the same hospital in Niigata where Japan's first HIV-positive patient received lentinan, the counteraction of chronic fatigue syndrome was equally successful. In Japan, the syndrome was originally dubbed "immune depression disease" or IDD, and at the time (1985) it seemed that Japan, if not the entire world, was witnessing a new kind of immune nightmare.

The symptoms of less than half the normal level of natural killer cell activity, "uncomfortable dullness," and "unexplained fever" persisting for several years[1] are today only too familiar to chronic fatigue syndrome patients in the Western world. But at the time, this was something new to the Japanese, or so it seemed. The main immunologic feature of IDD later resulted in the name change to "low natural killer syndrome" or LNKS,[2] which is identical to chronic fatigue syndrome (CFS) here.[3, 4] Before the practice of checking for NK activity, which has now become standard by CFS researchers internationally, some LNKS patients were occasionally treated by psychiatrists, because they suffered from depression and at the time there were no other clear-cut symptoms to go on, the same dilemma CFS patients have endured.

In 1985 Dr. Tadao Aoki of the Shinrakuen Hospital first reported that in an undisclosed number of LNKS patients lentinan injections (1 mg/day, every other day) resulted in rapid improvement of the "dullness." There was also a gradual return of body temperature and of NK activity to normal levels. Complete recovery in the majority of patients took only a few months.[5]

Two years later, Dr. Aoki and the world's authority on NK cells, Dr. Ronald

B. Herberman of the Pittsburgh Cancer Institute, reported on twenty-three Japanese patients. They ranged in age from fourteen to seventy-seven, but most were under forty and had presented chronic LNKS symptoms of long-standing duration, some for over twenty years. The treatment with lentinan required six months or more to bring their NK activity to within a normal range. In a few weeks, however, fevers vanished and the feeling of "well-being" returned. Aoki cautioned that even though a patient feels normal after two weeks on lentinan, stopping the treatment at that time results in nearly all the symptoms returning. Even so, the full dose can be gradually reduced after a few months.[6]

Seven patients experienced headaches, dizziness, or both. Every patient was beset with fatigue, "uncomfortable dullness," exhaustion, a decrease in physical and mental interests, and a fever resistant to any conventional treatment. Aoki and Herberman also noticed LNKS symptoms of lesser frequency, including anorexia, arthralgia, arthritis, pharyngitis, "nervous system symptoms," myalgia (muscle pains), and cervical lymph node swelling. Some of these patients had previously been treated with drugs for depression by psychiatrists who thought surely they were dealing with neurotics and depressives.[7] But for Dr. Aoki, who routinely treated AIDS and cancer patients with lentinan, the symptoms of fatigue and dullness were all too familiar and had often abated with lentinan.[8, 9] Moreover, in healthy people he found lentinan prevented exhaustion from "overwork."[10]

Lentinan has the same "effective activity" given orally as it does by injection.[11] During a visit to the U.S. National Institutes of Health in 1986, Dr. Aoki explained that the fifty-nine patients he had treated for LNKS showed great improvement in their NK cell counts when, as outpatients, they followed up with lentinan orally as a maintenance drug. Hospital costs were reduced, and the nasty business of needles was avoided altogether. For oral use, the amount was increased to 5 mg, which is five times the intravenous dose.[12]

The amount of lentinan in the fruit-body of the mushroom is actually rather small (0.88 to 1.17 mg per 6 to 8 grams of mushroom),[13] though lentinan is not the only polysaccharide responsible for the immunoactivity of the mushroom.[14] However, the best and most convenient products are concentrated extracts of shiitake, whether of the mycelium, the fruit-body, or both, since a gram of extract can equal 2 or even 10 grams of dried mushroom. Shiitake extracts are available in many health food stores in North America, western Europe, and most of the Orient.

Proposing yet another name for the disease, Chronic Fatigue Immune Dysfunction Syndrome (CFIDS), "since immune dysfunction appears to be a hallmark of the disease process," researchers Nancy L. Eby and colleagues from the Pittsburgh Cancer Institute found NK cell activity lower in symptomatic cases than in nonsymptomatic cases.[15] The "most consistent" abnormal reading of the immune system she has found is "very low" NK cell activity.[16] Although as much as a 50 percent lower than normal NK cell activity has sometimes been reported in major depression and in cases of severe stress,[17–19] low-NK cell activity now appears consistent among CFS patients.[20–23]

THE STRESS OF CFS

The typical CFS patient suffers with a bizarre range of symptoms.[24] Most do recover, but at least 1 percent may go on to have the disease for the rest of their lives.[25] The typical patient may endure years of mental confusion, muscle pains, crushing fatigue, headaches, earaches, irregular heartbeat, hair loss, joint aches, forgetfulness, tinnitus, swollen glands, night sweats, and insomnia. All the while, these symptoms will fluctuate, being at times slight and at other times incapacitating—more than enough to keep the patient from working, and that alone has destroyed lives.[26]

Few are in agreement on the real cause of CFS, but everyone concedes that stress or distress is an important factor. A follow-up questionnaire given to patients admitted to a British hospital with "unexplained fatigue," revealed that the majority of 144 cases (69 percent) complained of sleep problems. And although 94 percent thought some kind of infection had caused their illness, 67 percent believed stress had been a part of the cause.[27]

Depression is diagnosed in 50 to 80 percent of CFS cases,[28] but there are some striking differences in these patients when compared to depressives. The U.S. National Institutes of Mental Health, following almost four years of tests, reported that CFS patients consistently show a hormonal imbalance the opposite of what patients with major depression show. CFS patients have low levels of a steroid hormone known as cortisol and increased ACTH, a pituitary hormone. Conversely, depressives have high levels of cortisol and low levels of ACTH. The pituitary secretes ACTH (adrenocorticotropic hormone), which in turn stimulates the adrenals to secrete cortisol, especially in times of stress. Insufficient cortisol production is characterized by swollen lymph nodes, feverishness, disturbances in mood and sleep, a worsening of allergic reactions, joint pains (arthralgias), muscle pains (myalgias), and fatigue following exercise,[29] all of which are symptoms of CFS.[30]

Along with low NK cell activity, a depressed level of helper T-cells is now one of the diagnostic criteria for CFS.[31] Depressives show either an increased[32] or a decreased number of helper T-cells.[33] (Although by itself this is not a decisive criterion to distinguish CFS from depression, the question naturally arising from this observation is just how many patients diagnosed with depression have in fact had cases of CFS. No one knows.) Even though private researchers had been making similar findings for some years, a lower than normal helper T-cell count was finally established in CFS patients by the National Institute of Allergy and Infectious Diseases (NIAID) only in 1992. This represented the first time government scientists acknowledged that CFS was a real immune "dysfunction."[34]

Ranging in age from twenty-four to forty-nine, the five men and thirteen women with CFS studied by NIAID were all too sick to work full time. Only six worked at all. For seventeen of these patients, the disease started "abruptly with an infectious-type episode." The NIAID researchers had to admit that the abnormally low lymphocyte responsiveness in these patients lent credence to many private studies that had already found a host of immunologic abnormalities in patients with the disease. But the biggest breakthrough in the NIAID study concerned the helper T-cell.[35, 36]

Normally, these cells circulate in our bloodstream unchanged, or "naïve," until they encounter antigen, the bit of intelligence from a virus or other pathogen that immune cells use to recognize intruders. Then they become "memory" T-cells that remember the antigen they encountered when reexposed to it and stimulate other immune cells to attack. When this occurs, molecular receptors on their surface undergo a chemical change. It seems that this process can also occur without a pathogen, for in depressives the number of memory T-cells is higher than normal and higher than in people with CFS.[37] It is as if the immune system of depressives anticipated being attacked, which in some ways is not inconsistent with the character of the typical depressive.

The NIAID scientists found that not only are there fewer detectable naive T-cells in the bloodstream of CFS patients, their memory T-cells, although at normal levels, have a greater than normal number of adhesion molecules on the surface. These molecules allow the T-cells in the bloodstream to detect and to attach themselves to various tissues, which is where the missing naive T-cells appear to have gone. That implies that somewhere along the way, they changed to adhering memory cells. What could have caused that? The NIAID scientists speculated that neurohormonal, neuropsychiatric, or infectious agents could be the underlying cause. They further suggest that tender lymph nodes and the joint and muscle pains so common in CFS could be the result of cytokines (interleukins, interferons, and others) excreted by the immune cells in the tissues where they adhere, for it is well known that those molecules cause inflammation. They note that just such a scenario is found in inflammatory bowel disease.[38] It was no surprise to learn that 80 percent of CFS patients have some degree of irritable bowel syndrome,[39, 40] a disorder held as being of psycho-physiologic origin.

Much to their credit, the NIAID researchers included a group of chronically fatigued patients for comparison. Although their debilitating and prolonged fatigue began after an acute infectious illness, their number of symptoms fell short of the Centers for Disease Control and Prevention criteria for true CFS. Either they were able to maintain a level of daily activity greater than 50 percent of what normal people perform, or they only had four to seven of the symptoms needed to qualify, or both. Nevertheless, they showed immune cell changes similar to those the NIAID team had just found in CFS patients,[41] indicating the CDCP definition of CFS may be unduly limited. All these findings seem to speak volumes for the use of a T-cell stimulant such as lentinan in CFS, for it appears that lentinan and other immunostimulants mimicking antigens occupy the attention of the tissue-embedded T-cells sufficient to distract them from their lairs.

Mental stress can lower our levels of helper T-cells, and emotional stress, from a difficult marriage or from caring for terminally ill family members, for example, can lower numbers of NK cells as well as helper T-cells.[42, 43] And because repeated stress can lower NK cell activity and interferon production,[44-46] the likelihood of viral infections increases with long-term stress. When one adds loneliness, major depression, too many day-to-day hassles, and stressful events—every one of which has been tied to the incidence of low NK cell activity[47]—discerning the possible causes of this immune abnormality in CFS becomes extremely challenging.

It is well known that repeated stress, which results in chronic stress, can also produce depression. An estimate by the U.S. President's Commission on Mental Health gave 25 percent as the number of people in the United States in need of professional mental care, and 25 percent as the number experiencing the degree of stress known to produce anxiety and depression.[48] And that was in the 1970s! Rather than stimulate research, however, these facts have only helped to confuse CFS with depression. Clearly, they are not the same. Even psychological assessments of CFS patients reveal a definite difference from depression.

Using the Minnesota Multiphasic Personality Inventory (MMPI), Linda Iger, Ph.D., uncovered some findings that will help to shed light on an otherwise dimly understood disease. While unique, the CFS psychological profile shows great similarity to one of "chronic illness," with concerns focused on bodily health. Female patients have considerable amounts of distress, indications of significant depression, and fears of a "complete physiological breakdown." These fears may not be unsubstantiated. Dr. Iger warns, "It is important to note that others with profiles similar to this *do* experience physiological breakdown in middle to late age as a result of continuous autonomic nervous system arousal, which may be the result of processing stress physiologically, rather than through the emotions." (The autonomic nervous system is the part that regulates the actions of smooth muscles, glands, and heart muscle.) She concludes that the CFS patient is probably "in a constant state of tension and anxiety."[49]

SUSPECTS IN THE SYNDROME

Many physicians still believe the syndrome is a form of depression; never mind that CFS is now an officially recognized illness by no less than the U.S. National Institutes of Health.[50] Close to 85 percent of patients recall the day they came down with the disease, usually following a viral infection.[51] How many have it? That question only began to be answered in 1992. The Centers for Disease Control and Prevention are now looking into the matter with investigators at research stations in major cities across the United States. Perhaps in a few years we will have a clear idea of the real number of people affected.[52] The experts are saying, conservatively, that over one million Americans have the disease.[53] How many will eventually be diagnosed is difficult to estimate, but five times the one million or so known cases would be reasonable.

Looking for a cause of the disease, researchers from Australia, the United States, and Britain have probed a veritable menagerie of viruses.[54–59] So far, however, there is no collective agreement that any one virus is the cause of CFS. Human herpesvirus 6 (HHV-6), a different virus from herpes simplex I or II, continues to be a main suspect, partly for the reason that CFS patients have often shown signs of an active infection with this virus.[60] Previously associated with helper T-cell deficiencies,[61] this suspect is made all the more ominous with the recent discovery that HHV-6 can not only infect NK cells but can also kill them. According to the National Cancer Institute, the evidence suggests that this virus has the potential to actually suppress the body's "natural anti-viral immunity."[62] HHV-6 is known to cause a febrile disease in infants, who show symptoms reminiscent of CFS. In young children, HHV-6 causes exanthema subitum,[63] which produces a high fever for seventy-two to ninety-six hours; prior to the fever falling or soon after, a raised rash appears and spreads from the torso to other areas.[64] Among other illnesses, HHV-6 is suspected as a cofactor in hepatitis[65] and appears to cause a severe infectious-mononucleosis–like syndrome.[66]

Next to HHV-6, the latest of possible suspects to show up in the United States is an HTLV-II–*like* virus.[67] Let me emphasize here that this is only *like* HTLV-II and not the same entity. HTLV-II appears to have the same disease potential as its relative, HTLV-I, the leukemia virus noted in the last chapter.

Version II is now epidemic in AIDS patients across the United States, although largely in intravenous drug users.[68] Oddly, HTLV-II appears to infect women twice as often as men.[69]

Commenting on the viral factor in CFS, Byron Hyde, M.D., of the Nightingale Research Foundation in Ottawa, explains that there are presently two camps: "One is that the viral infection becomes persistent due to a derangement, breakdown, or non-effectiveness of the normal immune mechanism. Another school simply believes that the observed apparent immune dysregulation is related to the effects of a persisting chronic viral infection or the persistence of a viral fragment that triggers an abnormal immune response."[70]

TREATMENTS FOR CFS

Many CFS patients are taking a host of herbal and other natural medications, and some feel much better when they include the mycelial extract of shiitake.[71] One of the first signs of improvement is when the symptoms stop their wanton fluctuations.[72] Some patients get by on 400 mg a day.[73] Others require 1,800 mg a day.[74] There are many testimonies to the benefits of the extract in CFS,[75, 76] which is now one of the most frequently used supplements by people with CFS.[77] One company in the United States sends profits from the sale of LEM and other natural products to scientists dedicated to unravelling the nature of this baffling disease. The same concern has raised more funds for CFS research than any other organization.[78]

Unlike Ampligen, a costly interferon-inducing drug currently being tested against the syndrome,[79] the mycelium contains lentinan[80] and a host of antitumor,[81] antiviral, and otherwise immunoactive substances. In addition, the mycelial extract contains riboflavin (vitamin B_2), thiamine (vitamin B_1), complexes of polysaccharides and proteins, and nucleic acid derivatives.[82, 83] Yet it also contains an interferon-inducer in the form of KS-2.[84–91] Blood samples from cancer patients on KS-2 showed a very definite antiviral action,[92] and in mice given KS-2 orally in small doses—as little as 2 mg/kg—serum levels of interferon increased fortyfold.[93] The dried mycelium contains over 1 mg of pure KS-2 per gram. In a less than purified form, KS-2 occurs at about 5.6 mg per gram of dried mycelium; even in that form there was strong activity when it was taken orally: 20 mg/kg induced a high level of interferon, and 1 mg/kg produced antitumor activity in mice.[94]

Regrettably, at the time of this writing no one was conducting clinical trials with LEM or with lentinan against what is undeniably a very serious disease. This fact is made even more lamentable when both these shiitake by-products are known to restore NK cell activity. Whether LEM would benefit the patient with major depression who shows low NK cell activity also remains to be studied. The problem is simply one of cost. Some prominent physicians in the field have made proposals for larger, more controlled clinical studies of shiitake products than found in the few pilot studies to date, but obtaining funds is extremely difficult.[95, 96]

We may be grateful for at least one study of the mycelial extract in CFS. It was a small preliminary study by Jay A. Goldstein, M.D., director of the CFS Institute in Anaheim Hills, California. From it he found LEM definitely merits further investigation. Dr. Goldstein had tried a veritable "laundry list" of immunomodulators against CFS without success.[97] But with LEM, he was "impressed" that around 30 percent of the patients felt "better" and about half felt "considerably better." Only a couple of patients felt worse. Goldstein added that the improvements found appeared to be overall, which, he has noticed, is true for other kinds of "effective" immunomodulators used to treat this disease.[98]

If there is one aspect to this disease that more than any other is preventing people from getting better, it has got to be misdiagnosis. But then all that most physicians have relied on are symptoms; any biochemical markers have yet to be agreed on. Medications present their own set of problems. They seem best tolerated when taken in low doses at first and never abruptly stopped: starting low, weaning slow. Another rule of thumb is that typically some things seem to work for a time and then fail, with the patient back to square one, or perhaps one and a half.[99] From the few clinical studies performed to date, the best results are from magnesium sulphate injections (intramuscular),[100] evening primrose oil (essential fatty acids),[101, 102] Ampligen (polyribonucleotide),[103] Kutapressin (polypeptides),[104] lentinan,[105] schizophyllan or SPG (a polysaccharide),[106] and nucleic acid derivatives (adenosine compounds).[107–110]

All of these substances require repeated studies with larger numbers of patients and controls to be judged for effectiveness. Among these natural products, SPG merits further mention for it has much in common with lentinan.

SCHIZOPHYLLAN

Schizophyllan, or SPG, is chemically related to lentinan and has a similar structure. SPG is derived from the mycelium of suehirotake, a small fan-shaped mushroom (*Schizophyllum commune*) that appears like little shells of white lace.[111] Extremely common on old wooden planks, it also grows on trees and deadwood in many parts of the world.[112] Most mushroom books list it as far too tough to be edible, but in Africa people get around that by boiling it for an hour or two in water with vegetable salt. When dried, the mushroom contains 17 percent protein.[113] In Mexico, the fungus is called *chiquito* and is a highly praised food, which is fried with sesame and beans or cooked.[114] In traditional Chinese medicine, the "fan fungus" is stewed with eggs to provide a tonic to strengthen the body and "effectively" cure leukorrhea[115] and "gynecological diseases" in general.[116]

Also known as sizofiran, SPG is one of a large number of structurally related polysaccharides known as beta-glucans. Now a product of Kaken Pharmaceutical of Tokyo, it has shown immunologic activities in animals and benefits to cancer patients similar to that of lentinan.[117–119] True to its roots in folk medicine, for gynecological diseases SPG is now largely used in the treatment of cervical cancer.[120–123]

In the spring of 1992, Dr. Atsushi Uchida of Kyoto University announced that he had tested the glucan in eleven Japanese CFS patients, and ten had clearly shown improvements. Of these, three were able to return to work. The other seven, who were so ill they couldn't even maintain household chores or walk up a flight of stairs, all had resumed a "regular life." For all ten, NK cell activity levels were restored to "normal."[124]

By the summer of 1993, Dr. Uchida had treated over thirty patients with SPG, some of them Americans and Canadians. About half of them had made a complete recovery from the disease for over six months and were living a normal life.[125] These patients had had severe cases. Before SPG, they had been largely confined to home. Whatever treatment they had received previously was without any effect in improving their symptoms. But after one to two months of SPG daily (20 mg a day, orally), for more than 90 percent, the debilitating fatigue was either reduced or entirely gone, without any side effects from the treatment. NK cell activity was restored in consistent parallel to the abatement of symptoms.[126] It is interesting to note that as with patients with major depression,[127] there were signs of an overactive immune system. For example, the rate at which lymphocytes were produced in the blood was elevated, but after treatment the rate normalized.[128]

Serum levels of interleukin 2 were also elevated, returning to normal after SPG. Elevated levels of interleukin 2 receptor-bearing cells would tend to indicate immune system activation, since these receptors are found on the membrane of T-cells in an activated state. However, the responsiveness of T-cells to activations by interleukin 2 only returned in the CFS patients after therapy with SPG.[129] It is interesting to note that patients with major depression also show a higher than normal level of interleukin 2.[130]

One of the body's own immunostimulants, interleukin 2 is a protein the immune system uses to activate antibody-producing cells to make more antibodies, to activate NK cells to produce gamma-interferon, and to stimulate T-cells to make more interleukin 2. The protein is best known as a T-cell stimulant and experimental agent in new cancer and AIDS therapies, and for treatment of resistant tuberculosis.[131–133] In a healthy person, interleukin 2 causes NK cells to become active.

Dr. Uchida found that interleukin 2 receptors on the NK cells of CFS patients were normal; only, as if distracted, the NK cells would not respond to the interleukin 2 signals to become active. After SPG, those responses normalized.[134] You may recall from the previous chapter that a similar situation involving T-cells and antigens with impaired immunologic memory is now proposed in AIDS.

With SPG, the greatest improvements were found with an 80 to 90 percent reduction in frequency of chronic fatigue, swollen lymph nodes, sore muscles, neuropsychological problems, and pharyngitis. After-exercise fatigue became slight in about 50 percent of patients, and around

50 percent no longer suffered from high irritability, muscle aches, chills and fevers, swollen lymph nodes, pharyngitis, sore throats, headaches, confusion, depression, poor sleep, thinking difficulties, and poor concentration.[135] Outside of Japan, the availability of SPG will depend on a lengthy process of drug approval and testing.

Dr. Byron Hyde, a world authority on CFS, doesn't advocate any treatment just yet.[136] He says, "There are many folk remedies, vitamins, amino acids and other treatments that are not dangerous." Even though no scientific validation of their effectiveness is known to him, he is open-minded enough to state that they may help to alleviate symptoms, "or the disease."[137]

Hyde points to descriptions of CFS from the distant past, indicating one that exists in the Ebers papyrus and would place the disease in 1900 B.C., if not earlier.[138] If that is indeed the case, then, as more than one authority has suggested, we may be wise to investigate potions and herbs from the past,[139] for CFS may have already been cured in some traditional system of folk medicine in which the same disease was or still is known but under a different name.[140]

While he knew shiitake had beneficial effects on the immune system, Kisaku Mori was an adamant proponent of shiitake as a *blood* tonic. He made numerous references to the concept of a *toning* action by shiitake, often by citing small clinical studies conducted at Japanese universities during the early 1970s. Mori reported that the blood congestion in the brain that causes insomnia may be alleviated by eating shiitake regularly. And for cold extremities (hands and feet), fatigue, hemorrhoids, acid stomach, ulcers, kidney diseases, low blood pressure, high blood pressure, sexual weakness, arthritis, nasal polyps, disease-related blindness, nearsightedness, pyorrhea, leukemia, poor complexion, neuralgia (pain along a nerve), or "the color of the blood," he knew people, including physicians, who claimed great improvements from eating shiitake or from taking a shiitake extract.[141] The fact that so many of these problems appear in CFS patients should lead the investigator in search of new CFS drugs to take a serious look at shiitake. As you can see from the following partial list of symptoms and their estimated frequency of occurrence in CFS, many of the same problems Mori cites commonly attend this syndrome:[142–146]

Insomnia (90–98%)
Fatigue (95–100%)
Ulcers
Low blood pressure (86%)
Transient blindness
Dry mouth (30–40%)
Arthralgias (80%)

Cold extremities (65%)
Heartburn (40%)
Very tender kidneys (40%)
Low libido (10–30%)
Blurred vision (40–60%)
Poor complexion (20–25%)
Myalgias (91%)

TABLE 4

SHIITAKE'S ACTIVE CONSTITUENTS[147–167]

CONSTITUENT	ACTION	PART	SOURCE
Nucleoside or nucleic acid derivatives	Platelet aggregation inhibitory	Fruit-body	147
Eritadenine (amino acid)	Hypolipedemic (cholesterol lowering); normalizing effect on bile acid ratio in liver	Fruit-body	148, 149
Sulphide	Antifungal	Fruit-body	150
C-1-2 (polysaccharide)	Immunoactive	Mycelium	151
Lectin	Immunoactive	Fruit-body	152
Lentinan (polysaccharide)	Immunoactive	Fruit-body Mycelium	153–157
Emitanin (polysaccharide)	Immunoactive	Mycelium	158
EP3 (lignin)	Antiviral, immunoactive	Mycelium	159, 160
KS-2, KS-2-B (peptidomannans)	Antiviral, immunoactive, antibacterial	Mycelium	161–163

CONSTITUENT	ACTION	PART	SOURCE
Double-stranded RNA (polyribonucleotides)	Immunoactive	Fruit-body, mycelium, spores	164, 165
Ac2P (polysaccharide)	Antiviral	Fruit-body	166
FBP (protein)	Antiviral (plant viruses)	Fruit-body	167
Thioproline (TCA) (amino acid)	Nitrite scavenger	Fruit-body	168

Endnotes

CHAPTER ONE

1. K. Mori, *Mushrooms As Health Foods* (Tokyo: Japan Publications, 1974), 24–26.
2. B. Liu and Y.-S. Bau, *Fungi Pharmacopoeia (Sinica)* (Oakland, Calif.: Kinoko Company, 1980), 108.
3. British Columbia Ministry of Agriculture, *Chinese Mushroom Feasibility Study,* Project No. 271043 (Vancouver, B.C., 1979).
4. W. M. Breene, "Nutritional and Medicinal Value of Speciality Mushrooms," *Journal of Food Protection* 53 (1990): 883–94.
5. M. Kanetani, "Mushroom in Manufacture of Fermented Milk Products," *Japanese Patent* 02,283,240, November 20, 1990, in *Chemical Abstracts* 114 (1991): 450 (C.A. 114: 100176c).
6. *Bon Appétit* magazine, April 1990, 22, 62, and 118. For the restaurant industry, a video about shiitake ("Shiitake Mushrooms: Cooking American with an Oriental Favorite") is available from SHII-GAW, Shiitake Growers Association of Wisconsin, P.O. Box 99, Birchwood, Wisconsin 54817. I would also highly recommend the cookbook by Jennifer Snyder, *The Shiitake Way* (The Book Publishing Co., Summertown, Tenn., 1993).
7. S. T. Chang, "Mushrooms As Human Food," *BioScience* 30 (1980): 399–401.
8. Ibid.
9. L. Wang et al., "Analysis of Amino Acid Content of 30 Varieties of Edible Fungi," *Mushroom Journal of the Tropics* 10 (1990): 74–78.
10. J. Timmer et al., "A Nutritional Analysis and Development of Promotional Materials for Shiitake Mushroom Producers in Wisconsin," *Shiitake News* 7 (1990): 6–11.
11. M. Imake et al., "Study on Digestibility and Energy Availability of Daily Food Intake (Part 4 *Shiitake Mushroom*)," *Japanese Journal of Hygiene* 46 (1991): 905–12 (in Japanese).
12. See note 7 above.
13. See note 10 above.

14. T. Kobayashi et al., "Shiitake and Vitamin D," *Vitamins* (Kyoto) 62 (1988): 483–90 (in Japanese).

15. See note 10 above.

16. P. Millet et al., "Nutrient Intake and Vitamin Status of Healthy French Vegetarians and Nonvegetarians," *American Journal of Nutrition* 50 (1989): 718–27.

17. T. Ito, "Cultivation of *Lentinus edodes,*" in *Edible Mushrooms*, eds., S.T. Chang and W. A. Hayes (Academic Press, 1978), 461–73.

18. P. Przybillowicz and J. Donaghue, *Shiitake Grower's Handbook* (Dubuque, Iowa: Kendall Hunt Publishing, 1991).

19. See note 1 above.

20. T. Matsumotto and K. Tokimoto, "Quantitative Changes of Bioelements During Fruitbody Development in *Lentinus edodes,*" *Reports of the Tottori Mycological Society,* no. 25 (1987): 62–67 (in Japanese).

21. H. Yokokawa, "Analyses of General and Inorganic Components and Fatty Acid Compositions of Fruit Bodies of Higher Fungi," *Transactions of the Mycological Society of Japan* 25 (1984): 531–37.

22. S. T. Chang, "Mushrooms As Human Food," *BioScience* 30 (1980): 399–401.

23. H. Yoshida et al., "Changes in Carbohydrates and Organic Acids During Development of Mycelia and Fruit-Bodies of Shiitake Mushroom *Lentinus edodes* Berk. Sing," *Journal of the Japan Society of Food Science and Technology* 34 (1987): 274–81 (in Japanese).

24. C. Li and X. Kue, "Analysis and Comparison of Amino Acid Content in Fungal Mycelia and Fermentation Broth," *Nanjing Daxue Xuebao, Ziran Kexue* 23 (1987): 442–52 (in Chinese).

25. T. Kobayashi et al., "Shiitake and Vitamin D," *Vitamins* (Kyoto) 62 (1988): 438–90 (in Japanese).

26. M. Hasiguchi et al., "Composition of Foods: Vegetables and Vegetable Products" in *USDA Agricultural Handbook,* nos. 8–11 (1984): 231–32.

27. E. V. Crisan and A. Sands, "Nutritional Value," in *Edible Mushrooms*, eds., S. T. Chang and W. A. Hayes (Academic Press, 1978), 137–68.

28. See note 26 above.

29. See note 18 above.

30. D. J. Royse, "Effect of Spawn Run Time and Substrate Nutrition on Yield and Size of the Shiitake Mushroom," *Mycologia* 77 (1985): 756–62.

31. W. Yun-Chang, "Mycology in Ancient China," *The Mycologist* 21, part 2 (1987): 59–61.

32. See note 18 above.

33. K. Dionis, "Mushrooms from Trees," *Mushroom News* 38 (August 1990): 6–11.

34. J. Eden, introductory letter (1985), Forest Resource Centre, Route 2, Box 156A, Lanesboro, MN 55949; publishers of *Shiitake News*, a must read for growers.

35. Editorial, "On the Main Stem—Around the Nation," *Mushroom News* 38 (August 1990): 2–4.

36. See note 34 above.

37. Editorial, *Shiitake News* 9, no. 1 (1992): 10.

38. S. T. Chang and P. G. Miles, "A New Look at Cultivated Mushrooms," *BioScience* 34 (1984): 358–62.

39. Editorial, "Dancing Mushrooms," *Mushroom News* 38 (August 1990): 12–13.

CHAPTER TWO

1. B. Liu and Y.-S. Bau, *Fungi Pharmacopoeia (Sinica)* (Oakland, Calif.: Kinoko Company, 1980), 105–9.

2. K. Mori, *Mushrooms As Health Foods* (Tokyo: Japan Publications, 1974), 29–31.

3. F. Mayuzumi et al., "Bath Preparations Containing Mushroom Polysaccharides," *Japanese Patent* 61,129,113, June 17, 1986, in *Chemical Abstracts* 105 (1986): 361 (C.A. 105: 158629h).

4. Noda Shokkin Kogyo K. K., "Therapeutic Agents for Skin Diseases," *Japanese Patent* 58,180,428, October 21, 1983, in *Chemical Abstracts* 100 (1984): 351 (C.A. 100: 33273c).

5. *The Journal: Have a Talk with Owners,* January 1982, 18–23 (Tokyo monthly magazine in Japanese, translated).

6. H. Yahara, *Shukan Gedai (Weekly Magazine Today)*, Tokyo, December 17, 1983, 219–22 (in Japanese, translated).

7. N. Claydon, "Secondary Metabolic Products of Selected Agarics," in *Developmental Biology of Higher Fungi*, symposium of the British Mycological Society, University of Manchester, April 1984, eds., D. Moore et al. (Cambridge: Cambridge University Press, 1985), 561–79.

8. P.-G. Xiao et al., "Immunological Aspects of Chinese Medicinal Plants As Antiaging Drugs," *Journal of Ethnopharmacology* 38 (1993): 167–75.

9. Y. Sugi, *Seijikai (Political World)*, Tokyo, September 1981, 66–68 (in Japanese, translated).

10. T. Ito, "Cultivation of *Lentinus edodes*," in *Edible Mushrooms*, eds., S. T. Chang and W. A. Hayes (Academic Press, 1978), 461–73.

11. Y.-C. Wang, "Mycology in China with Emphasis on Review of the Ancient Literature," *Acta Mycologica Sinica* 4 (1985): 133–40.

12. See note 9 above.

13. See note 10 above.

14. H. C. Lu, *Chinese System of Food Cures: Prevention and Remedies* (New York: Sterling Publishing, 1986), 14–20, 99–100, 178, 182.

15. M. Ueno, ed., *Shokumotsu Honzo Bon Taisei*, vol. 5 (Kyoto: Rinsen Shoten, 1980), 284–85.

16. See note 9 above.
17. See note 10 above.
18. See note 9 above.
19. Mori, *Mushrooms As Health Foods*, 56.
20. Ibid., 43.
21. K. W. Cochran et al., "Botanical Sources of Influenza Inhibitors," *Antimicrobial Agents and Chemotherapy* (1966): 515–20.
22. A. Tsunoda and N. Ishida, "A Mushroom Extract As an Interferon Inducer," *Annals of the New York Academy of Sciences* 173 (1970): 719–26.
23. K. Mori and K. Mori, "Studies on the Virus-like Particles in *Lentinus edodes* (Shii-ta-ke)," in *Mushroom Science IX* (Part I), proceedings of the Ninth International Scientific Congress on the Cultivation of Edible Fungi, Tokyo, 1974 (Kiryu, Japan: Mushroom Research Institute, 1976), 541–56.
24. M. Takehara et al., "Antiviral and Antitumor Activities of Certain Double-Stranded Polyribonucleotides," *ICRM Annals* 3 (1983): 81–88.
25. M. Takehara et al., "Antitumor Effect of Virus-Like Particles from *Lentinus edodes* (Shiitake) on Ehrlich Acsites Carcinoma in Mice," *Archives of Virology* 68 (1981): 297–301.
26. See note 24 above.
27. F. Suzuki et al., "Mushroom Extract As an Interferon Inducer. I. Biological and Physiochemical Properties of Spore Extracts of *Lentinus edodes*," in *Mushroom Science IX* (Part I), proceedings of the Ninth International Scientific Congress on the Cultivation of Edible Fungi, Tokyo, 1974 (Kiryu, Japan: Mushroom Research Institute, 1976), 509–19.
28. Ibid.
29. Y. Yamamura and K. W. Cochran, "A Selective Inhibitor of Myxoviruses from Shii-ta-ke (*Lentinus edodes*)," in *Mushroom Science IX* (Part I), proceedings of the Ninth International Scientific Congress on the Cultivation of Edible Fungi, Tokyo, 1974 (Kiryu, Japan: Mushroom Research Institute, 1976), 495–507.
30. See notes 1, 19, and 20 above.
31. See note 19 above.
32. Mori, *Mushrooms As Health Foods*, 20.
33. S. Tokuda et al., "Reducing Mechanism of Plasma Cholesterol by Shii-ta-ke," in *Mushroom Science IX* (Part I), proceedings of the Ninth International Scientific Congress on the Cultivation of Edible Fungi, Tokyo, 1974 (Kiryu, Japan: Mushroom Research Institute, 1976), 445–62.
34. S. Tokuda and T. Kaneda, "Effect of Shii-ta-ke Mushroom on Plasma Cholesterol Levels in Rats," in *Mushroom Science X* (Part II), proceedings of the Tenth International Congress on the Science and Cultivation of Edible Fungi, Bordeaux, France, 1978 (Point de la Maye, France: L'Institut National de la Recherche Agronomique, 1979), 793–96.

35. V. E. C. Ooi et al., "Protective Effects of Some Edible Mushrooms on Paracetamol-Induced Liver Injury," in *First International Conference on Mushroom Biology and Mushroom Products, August 23–26, 1993, Hong Kong, Program and Abstracts* (Hong Kong: Department of Biology, Chinese University of Hong Kong, 1993), abstr. P-2-13: 139.

36. N. Sugano et al., "Anticarcinogenic Actions of Water-Soluble and Alcohol-Insoluble Fractions from Culture Medium of *Lentinus edodes* Mycelia," *Cancer Letters* 17 (1982): 109–14.

37. Y. Mizoguchi et al., "Protection of Liver Cells Against Experimental Damage by Extract of Cultured *Lentinus edodes* Mycelia (LEM)," *Gastroenterologia Japonica* 22 (1987): 459–64.

38. H. Amagase, "Treatment of Hepatitis B Patients with *Lentinus edodes* Mycelium," *Excerpta Medica* (1987): 316–21.

39. "JDF Research Funding," *Juvenile Diabetes Foundation International* 9 (1988): 42–50.

40. A. S. Bansal et al., "Cellular and Humoral Immunity in Patients with Insulin-Dependent Diabetes," *The Lancet* 342 (July 24, 1993): 246.

41. M. B. A. Oldstone et al., "Virus Persists in *B* Cells of Islets of Langerhans and Is Associated with Chemical Manifestations of Diabetes," *Science* 224 (1984): 1440–43.

42. J.-W. Yoon et al., "Virus-Induced Diabetes Mellitus," *New England Journal of Medicine* 300 (1979): 1173–79.

43. J. Satoh et al., "Inhibition of Development of Insulin-Dependent (Type I) Diabetes Mellitus in Nonobese Diabetic Mice by TNF and TNF Inducers," *Igaku no Aymumi* 147 (1988): 63–64.

44. T. Sharon, *Information Summary: Lentinus edodes (Shiitake) Mycelial Extract.* LEM Survey Project, El Torro, Calif., March 13, 1989. 10 pp.

45. Nancy Deutsch, "Look Beyond Blood Sugar When Treating Diabetes," *The Medical Post* (November 2, 1993): 50.

46. See note 44 above.

47. Dan Hurley, "Diabetics in a Tight Spot," *Medical World News* (July 1993): 22–24, 26, 27.

48. See note 1 above.

49. See notes 37 and 38 above.

50. A. Ueda et al., "Allergic Contact Dermatitis in Shiitake (*Lentinus edodes* [Berk] Sing) Growers," *Contact Dermatitis* 26 (1992): 228–33.

51. K. Tarvainen et al., "Allergy and Toxicodermia from Shiitake Mushrooms," *Journal of the American Academy of Dermatology* 24 (1991): 64–66.

52. Y. J. L. Kamm et al., "Provocation Tests in Extrinsic Allergic Alveolitis in Mushroom Workers," *Netherlands Journal of Medicine* (1991): 59–64.

53. A. Cox et al., "Provocation Tests in Patients with Extrinsic Allergic Alveolitis

Working with the Mushroom Shii-take (*Lentinus edodes*)," *European Respiratory Journal* 1, suppl. 2 (1988): 296S.

54. T. Nakamura and A. Kobayashi, "Toxikodermie Durch den Speisepilz Shiitake (Lentinus edodes)," *Der Hautartz* 36 (1985): 591–93.
55. See note 1 above.
56. Ibid.
57. Ibid.

CHAPTER THREE

1. S. Suzuki and S. Ohshima, "Influence of Shii-ta-ke (*Lentinus edodes*) on Human Serum Cholesterol," in *Mushroom Science IX* (Part I), proceedings of the Ninth International Scientific Congress on the Cultivation of Edible Fungi, Tokyo, 1974 (Kiryu, Japan: Mushroom Research Institute, 1976), 463–67.
2. L. H. Kimura et al., "Inhibition of Platelet Aggregation by Low Dalton Compounds from Aqueous Diasylates of Edible Fungi," *Federation Proceedings* 40, part 2 (1981): 809.
3. Y. Hokama and J. L. R. Y. Hokama, "*In Vitro* Inhibition of Platelet Aggregation by Low Dalton Compounds from Aqueous Dialysates of Edible Fungi," *Research Communications in Chemical Pathology and Pharmacology* 31 (1981): 177–80.
4. M. H. Knisely et al., "Sludged Blood," *Science* 106 (1947): 431–40.
5. Ibid.
6. Y. Sugi, *Seijikai* (*Political World*), Tokyo, September 1981, 66–68 (in Japanese, translated).
7. T. Ito, "Cultivation of *Lentinus edodes*," in *Edible Mushrooms*, eds., S. T. Chang and W. A. Hayes (Academic Press, 1978), 461–73.
8. R. B. Devereux et al., "Whole Blood Viscosity As a Determinant of Cardiac Hypertrophy in Systemic Hypertension," *American Journal of Cardiology* 54 (1984): 592–95.
9. H. I. Bicher and A. M. Beemer, "Induction of Ischemic Myocardial Damage by Red Blood Cell Aggregation (Sludge) in the Rabbit," *Journal of Atherosclerosis Research* 7 (1967): 409–14.
10. N. Fetkovska et al., "Low-Density Lipoprotein Enhances Platelet Activation in Parallel with the Height of Blood Pressure," *Journal of Hypertension* 6, suppl. 4 (1988): S646–48.
11. R. Virag et al., "Is Impotence an Arterial Disorder?" *The Lancet*, January 26, 1985, 181–84.
12. S. J. Chapman et al., "Zinc Levels in *Volvariella volvacea* Fruit Bodies and Mycelium," in *First International Conference on Mushroom Biology and Mushroom Products, August 23–26, 1993, Hong Kong, Program and Abstracts* (Hong

Kong: Department of Biology, Chinese University of Hong Kong, 1993), abstr. P-2-44: 154.

13. N. Claydon, "Secondary Metabolic Products of Selected Agarics," in *Developmental Biology of Higher Fungi,* symposium of the British Mycological Society, University of Manchester, April 1984, eds., D. Moore et al. (Cambridge: Cambridge University Press, 1985), 561–79.

14. V. T. Flynn, "Is the Shiitake Mushroom an Aphrodisiac and Cause of Longevity?" in *Mushroom Science XIII,* proceedings of the 13th International Congress on the Science and Cultivation of Edible Fungi, Dublin, Ireland, September 1–6, 1991, ed., M. J. Maher (Rotterdam/Brookfield, Vt.: A.A. Balkema, 1991), 345–61.

15. T. F. Lue et al., "Functional Evaluation of Penile Arteries with Duplex Ultrasound in Vasodilator-Induced Erection," *Urologic Clinics of North America* 16 (1989): 799–807.

16. "Impotence: NIH Consensus Development Panel on Impotence," *Journal of the American Medical Association* 270 (1993): 83–90.

17. See note 12 above.

18. R. Lihva et al., "Antiatherosclerotic Properties of Higher Fungi. A Clinico-Experimental Study," *Voprosy Pitaniya* 1 (1989): 16–19 (in Russian).

19. L. H. Ryong et al., "Antiatherogenic and Antiatherosclerotic Effects of Mushroom Extracts Revealed in Human Aortic Intima Cell Culture," *Drug Development Research* 17 (1989): 109–18.

20. Ibid.

21. See note 18 above.

22. E. J. Lien, "Fungal Metabolites and Chinese Herbal Medicine As Immunostimulants," *Progress in Drug Research* 34 (1990): 395–420.

23. T. Willard and K. Jones, *Reishi Mushroom. Herb of Spiritual Potency and Medical Wonder.* Seattle: Sylvan Press, 1990.

24. M. Ueno, ed., *Shokumotsu Honzo Bon Taisei*, vol. 5. (Kyoto: Rinsen Shoten, 1980), 284–85.

25. See note 19 above.

26. Ibid.

27. Y. Kabir et al., "Effect of Shiitake (*Lentinus edodes*) and Maitake (*Grifola frondosa*) Mushrooms on Blood Pressure and Plasma Lipids of Spontaneously Hypertensive Rats," *Journal of Nutritional Sciences and Vitaminology* 33 (1987): 341–46.

28. Y. Kabir et al., "Dietary Effect of *Ganoderma lucidum* Mushroom on Blood Pressure and Lipid Levels in Spontaneously Hypertensive Rats (SHR)," *Journal of Nutritional Sciences and Vitaminology* 34 (1988): 433–38.

29. K. Kanmatsuse et al., "Studies on *Ganoderma lucidum*. I. Efficacy against Hypertension and Side Effects," *Yakugaku Zasshi* 105 (1985): 942–47.

30. K. Jones, "Reishi (*Ganoderma*): Longevity Herb of the Orient, Part One," *Townsend Letter for Doctors,* no. 117 (October 1992): 814–18.

31. See note 23 above.

32. Ibid.

33. S. Aung, "Medicinal Applications of Fungi and Fungal Secondary Metabolites with Emphasis on the Use of *Ling zhi* in Traditional Chinese Medicine," *Mushroom World* 3 (1992): 17–23.

34. See notes 2, 3, 18, 19, and 27 above.

35. T. Kaneda and S. Tokuda, "Effect of Various Mushroom Preparations on Cholesterol Levels in Rats," *Journal of Nutrition* 90 (1966): 371–76.

36. S. Tokuda et al., "Reducing Mechanism of Plasma Cholesterol by Shii-ta-ke," in *Mushroom Science IX* (Part I), proceedings of the Ninth International Congress on the Cultivation of Edible Fungi, Tokyo, 1974 (Kiryu, Japan: Mushroom Research Institute, 1976), 445–62.

37. S. Tokuda and T. Kaneda, "Effect of Shii-ta-ke Mushroom on Plasma Cholesterol Levels in Rats," in *Mushroom Science X* (Part II), proceedings of the Tenth International Congress on the Science and Cultivation of Edible Fungi, Bordeaux, France, 1978 (Point de la Maye, France: L'Institut National de la Recherche Agronomique, 1979), 793–96. See also S. Parthasarathy et al., *Biochemica et Biophysica Acta* 1044 (1990): 275–83, and M. I. Mackness et al., *Biochemical Journal* 294 (1993): 829–34.

38. See note 27 above.

39. S.-I. Kurasawa et al., "Studies on Dietary Fibre of Mushrooms and Edible Wild Plants," *Nutrition Reports International* 26 (1982): 167–73.

40. Ibid.

41. Y. Yamamura and K. W. Cochran, "Chronic Hypocholesterolemic Effect of *Lentinus edodes* in Mice and Absence of Effect on Scrapie," in *Mushroom Science IX* (Part I), proceedings of the Ninth International Scientific Congress on the Cultivation of Edible Fungi, Tokyo, 1974 (Kiryu, Japan: Mushroom Research Institute, 1976), 489–93. See also note 27 above.

42. M. Ohtsuru, "Anti-Obesity Activity by Orally Administered Powder of Maitake Mushroom *(Grifola frondosa)*." *Anshin*, Tokyo, July 1992, 198–200.

43. Ibid.

44. M. Yokota, "Observatory Trial of Anti-Obesity Activity of Maitake Mushroom *(Grifola frondosa)*." *Anshin*, Tokyo, July 1992, 202–3.

45. See note 42 above.

46. See note 44 above.

47. G. H. Lincoff, *The Audubon Society Field Guide to North American Mushrooms* (New York: Alfred A. Knopf, Chanticleer Press, 1981): 463, 474–75.

48. S. Wakita, "Thiamine-Destruction by Mushrooms," *Science Report of Tokohama National University* 2 (1976): 39–70. Besides maitake, various kinds of tea, including jasmine, black, and oolong teas, also have thiaminase activity. However, even in people with a thiamine-deficient diet, the destruction of thiamine from drinking tea is readily alleviated by a 10-mg thiamine supplement. See S. L. Vimokesant et al., "Effect of Tea Consumption on Thiamine Status in Man," *Nutrition Reports International* 9 (1974):371–76.

49. See note 1 above.

50. Ibid.

51. K. Mori, *Mushrooms As Health Foods* (Tokyo: Japan Publications, 1974), 62.

52. See note 1 above.

53. Ibid.

54. J. Stamler et al., "Is Relationship Between Serum Cholesterol and Risk of Premature Death from Coronary Heart Disease Continuous and Graded?" *Journal of the American Medical Association* 256 (1986): 2823–28.

55. L. A. Simons, "Interrelations of Lipids and Lipoproteins With Coronary Artery Disease Mortality in 19 Countries," *American Journal of Cardiology* 57 (1986): 5G–10G.

56. S. M. Grundy, "Cholesterol and Coronary Heart Disease," *Journal of the American Medical Association* 256 (1986): 2849–58.

57. P. Van't Veer et al., "Dietary Fat and the Risk of Breast Cancer," *International Journal of Epidemiology* 19 (1990): 12–18.

58. "Diet Linked to Lung Cancer," *Globe and Mail*, Toronto, March 30, 1993, A5.

59. K. L. Erickson and N. E. Hubbard, "Dietary Fat and Immunity," in *Human Nutrition—A Comprehensive Treatise, vol. 8: Nutrition and Immunology*, D. M. Klurfeld, ed. (New York: Plenum Press, 1993), 51–78.

60. A. Berken and B. Benacerraf, "Depression of Reticuloendothelial System Phagocytic Function by Ingested Lipids," *Proceedings of the Society for Experimental Biology and Medicine* 128 (1968): 793–95.

61. R. H. Fiser et al., "Altered Immune Functions in Hypercholesterolemic Monkeys," *Infection and Immunity* 8 (1973): 105–9.

62. M. U. Dianzani et al., "The Influence of Enrichment with Cholesterol on the Phagocytic Activity of Rat Macrophages," *Journal of Pathology* 118 (1976): 193–99.

63. H. A. Chapman and J. B. Hibbs, "Modulation of Macrophage Tumoricidal Capability by Components of Normal Serum: A Central Role for Lipid," *Science* 197 (July 15, 1977): 282–85.

64. D. M. Klurfeld et al., "Alterations of Host Defenses Paralleling Cholesterol-Induced Atherogensis. II. Immunological Studies in Rabbits," *Journal of Medicine* 10 (1979): 49–64.

CHAPTER FOUR

1.   S. Reiser, "Metabolic Aspects of Nonstarch Polysaccharides," *Food Technology* (January 1984): 107–13.

2.   E. J. Lien, "Fungal Metabolites and Chinese Herbal Medicine As Immuno-stimulants," *Progress in Drug Research* 34 (1990): 395–419.

3.   E. J. Lien and H. Gao, "Higher Plant Polysaccharides and Their Pharmacological Activities," *International Journal of Oriental Medicine* 15 (1990): 123–40.

4.   Editorial, "Fungi," *The Lancet* (September 26, 1925): 660.

5.   P.-K. Tsung, "Anticancer and Immunostimulating Polysaccharides," *Oriental Healing Arts International Bulletin* 12 (1987): 1–10.

6.   B. Liu and Y.-S. Bau, *Fungi Pharmacopoeia (Sinica)* (Oakland, Calif.: Kinoko Company, 1980), 194–97.

7.   Y.-P. Yang and D.-C. Yueh, *A Brief Status of the Production of Medical Fungi in China* (Beijing: Institute of Materia Medica, Chinese Academy of Medical Sciences, undated).

8.   T. Ikekawa et al., "Antitumor Activity of Aqueous Extracts of Edible Mushrooms," *Cancer Research* 29 (1969): 734–35.

9.   Y. Yoshioka et al., "Studies on Antitumor Activity of Some Fractions from Basidiomycetes. I. An Antitumor Acidic Polysaccharide Fraction of *P. ostreatus* (Fr.) Quel.," *Chemical and Pharmaceutical Bulletin* 20 (1972): 1175–80.

10.   T. Ikekawa et al., "Studies on the Antitumor Activity of Polysaccharides from *Flammulina velutipes* (Curt. ex Fr.) Sing.," *Cancer Chemotherapy Reports* 57, part 1 (1973): 85–86.

11.   Y. Yoshioka et al., "Studies on Antitumor Polysaccharides of *Flammulina velutipes* (Curt. ex Fr.) Sing.," *Chemical and Pharmaceutical Bulletin* 21 (1973): 1772–76.

12.   H. Maruyama et al., "Antitumor Activity of *Sarcodon aspratus* (Berk.) S. Ito and *Ganoderma lucidum* (Fr.) Karst.," *Journal of Pharmacobio-Dynamics* 12 (1989): 118–23.

13.   M. Ueno, ed., *Shokumotsu Honzo Bon Taisei*, vol. 5 (Kyoto: Rinsen Shoten, 1980), 284–85.

14.   L. Réthy et al., "The Host's-Defense Increasing (antitumor) Activity of Polysaccharides Prepared from *Lentinus cyanthiformis*," *Annales Immunologiae Hungaricae* 21 (1981): 285–90.

15.   See note 8 above.

16.   K. Matsumoto, *The Mysterious Reishi Mushroom* (Santa Barbara, Calif.: Woodbridge Press Publishing, 1979), 43.

17.   T. Ikekawa et al., "Antitumor Activity of Aqueous Extracts of Edible Mushrooms," *Cancer Research* 29 (1969): 734–35.

18.   See note 8 above.

19. G. Chihara et al., "Fractionation and Purification of the Polysaccharides with Marked Antitumor Activity, Especially Lentinan, from *Lentinus edodes* (Berk.) Sing. (An Edible Mushroom)," *Cancer Research* 30 (1970): 2776–81.

20. L. Nikl et al., "Influence of Seven Immunostimulants on the Immune Response of Coho Salmon to *Aeromonas salmonicida*," *Diseases of Aquatic Organisms* 12 (1991): 7–12.

21. T. Yano et al., "Polysaccharide-Induced Protection of Carp, *Cyprinus caripo* L., Against Bacterial Infection," *Journal of Fish Diseases* 14 (1991): 577–82.

22. K. Yoneda et al., "Inhibition of Tumor Metastasis by a Glucan, Lentinan with Reference to Macrophage Activation," *Shikoku Acta Medica* 40 (1984): 473–78.

23. J. E. Byram et al., "Potentiation of *Schistosome* Granuloma Formation," *American Journal of Pathology* 94 (1979): 201–22.

24. A. A. Luderer and H. Weetall, eds., *Clinical Cellular Immunology* (Clifton, N.J.: Humana Press, 1982), 301, 303.

25. J. D.-E. Young and Z. A. Cohn, "How Killer Cells Kill," *Scientific American* (January 1988): 38–44.

26. B. R. Bloom, "Interferons and the Immune System," *Nature* 284 (1980): 593–95.

27. T. Taguchi et al., "Cooperative Phase Studies of Lentinan," in *Current Chemotherapy and Immunotherapy*, vol. 2, eds., P. Perti and G. G. Grassi (Washington, D.C.: American Society for Microbiology, 1982), 1210–11.

28. Clinical brochure, *Lentinan (Ajinomoto)* 1 mg: *A New Type of Anticancer Drug* (Tokyo: Ajinomoto Co., undated).

29. T. Aoki, "Lentinan," in *Immune Modulating Agents and Their Mechanisms*, eds., R. L. Fenishel and M. A. Chirgis (New York and Basel: Marcel Dekker, 1984), 66–77.

30. K. Haranaka et al., "Antitumor Activity of Recombinant Human Tumor Necrosis Factor in Combination with Hyperthermia, Chemotherapy, or Immunotherapy," *Journal of Biological Response Modifiers* 6 (1987): 379–91.

31. H. Shimizu et al., "Augmentation of Antitumor Effect of Recombinant Interleukin-2 Activated Killer Cells by the Administration of *rIL-2* and Lentinan," *Acta Obstetrica Gynaecologica* (Japan) 40 (1988): 1899–1900.

32. See note 30 above.

33. See note 31 above.

34. M. Suzuki et al., "Induction of Endogenous Lymphokine-Activated Killer Activity by Combined Administration of Lentinan and Interleukin 2," *International Journal of Immunopharmacology* 12 (1990): 613–23.

35. S. Arinaga et al., "Enhanced Production of Interleukin 1 and Tumor Necrosis Factor by Peripheral Monocytes after Lentinan Administration in Patients with

Gastric Carcinoma," *International Journal of Immunopharmacology* 14 (1992): 43–47.

36. Y. Y. Maeda et al., "Genetic Control of the Expression of Two Biological Activities of an Antitumor Polysaccharide, Lentinan," *International Journal of Immunopharmacology* 13 (1991): 977–86.

37. A. Saito, "Pharmaceuticals Containing Lentinan for Treatment of Bone Damage," *Japanese Patent* 63 17,828, January 25, 1988, in *Chemical Abstracts* 109 (1988): 395 (C.A. 101: 176355c).

38. J. Tsubochi et al., "Preventive and Therapeutic Formulations Containing Lentinan for Disseminated Intravascular Clotting," *Japanese Patent* 62 72,620, April 3, 1987, in *Chemical Abstracts* 107 (1987): 325 (C.A. 107: 28406p).

39. See note 29 above.

40. H. Yamada et al., "Dermatological Composition Based on an Aqueous Phase," *United States Patent* 5, 126,135, June 30, 1992.

41. T. Shiio et al., "Combination Use of Lentinan with X-Ray Therapy in Mouse Experimental Tumor System. Part 2. Combination Effect on MM102 Syngeneic Tumor," *Gan to Kagaku Ryoho* 15 (1988): 475–79 (in Japanese), in *Chemical Abstracts* 109: 16677f.

42. E. J. Lien, "The Use of Chinese Herbal Medicine in Cancer Prevention and Chemotherapy: A Survey," *Oriental Healing Arts Bulletin* 13 (1988): 59–68.

43. D.-T. Chu et al., "Immunotherapy with Chinese Medicinal Herbs. I. Immune Restoration of Local Xeonogeneic Graft-Versus-Host Reaction in Cancer Patients by Fractionated *Astragalus membranaceous in Vitro*," *Journal of Clinical and Laboratory Immunology* 25 (1988): 119–23. See also X. Yu-ling, "Traditional and Western Medicine Treatment of 211 Cases of Late Stage Lung Cancer," *Chinese Journal of Integrated Medicine* 13 (1993): 135, abstract in *Chinese Medical Journal* 106 (1993): 720.

44. C.-M. Wang et al., "Studies on Chemical Protectors Against Radiation. XXXV. Effects of Radioprotective Chinese Traditional Medicines on Radiation-Induced Lipid Peroxidation *in Vivo* and *in Vitro*," *Chemical and Pharmaceutical Bulletin* 40 (1992): 493–98.

45. M. A. Chirigos and M. L. Patchen, "Survey of Newer Biological Response Modifiers for Possible use in Radioprotection," *Pharmacology and Therapeutics* 39 (1988): 243–46.

46. Ibid.

47. J. Matsubara et al., "Promotion of a New Radioprotective Antioxidant Agent," in *AIP Conference Proceedings*, vol. 186. High-Energy Radiation Background in Space, Sanibel Island, Florida, 1987. Eds., A. C. Rester and J. I. Trombka (New York: American Institute of Physics, 1989), 434–41.

48. A. Kosaka et al., "Synergistic Action of Lentinan (LTN) with Endocrine Therapy

for Breast Cancer in Rats and Humans," *Gan to Kagaku Ryoho* 14 (1987): 516–22 (in Japanese), in *Chemical Abstracts* 106: 207327q.

49. J. Hasegawa et al., "Inhibition of Mitomycin C-Induced Sister-Chromatid Exchanges in Mouse Bone Marrow Cells by the Immunopotentiators Krestin and Lentinan," *Mutation Research* 226 (1989): 9–12.

50. T. Teguchi and Y. Kaneko, "Lentinan: An Overview of Experimental and Clinical Studies of Its Action Against Cancer," in *Proceedings of the Seventh Symposium on Host Defense Mechanisms Against Cancer,* Hakone, Japan, November 8–10, 1985. *Excerpta Medica*, International Congress Series No. 738: 221–29.

51. T. Teguchi et al., "Clinical Efficacy of Lentinan on Patients with Stomach Cancer," *International Journal of Immunopharmacology* 7 (1985): 331.

52. See note 27 above.

53. See note 50 above.

54. See note 51 above.

55. See note 50 above.

56. Ibid.

57. S. Marcovitch and Y. Keisara, "The Synergistic Tumorcidal Activity of Anticancer Drugs and Oxidative Burst-Triggered Macrophages," *Cancer Immunology Immunotherapy* 20 (1985): 205–8. See also notes 27 and 34 above.

58. S. Abe et al., "Combination Antitumor Therapy with Lentinan and Bacterial Lipopolysaccharide Against Murine Tumors," *Japanese Journal of Cancer Research* 73 (1982): 91–96.

59. Ibid.

60. See note 8 above.

61. F. Morishige, lecture, in *Becoming Healthy with Reishi,* vol. 3 (Tokyo: Kampo Iyaku Shimbun, Toyo-Igaku Sha Co., 1988), 12–20 (in Japanese, translated).

62. F. Morishige et al., in *Vitamins and Cancer: Human Cancer Prevention by Vitamins and Micronutrients*, eds., F. L. Meyskens and K. N. Prasad (Clifton, N.J.: Humana Press, 1980), 399–427.

63. See note 61 above.

64. C. Wiley, "The Medicinal Side of Mushrooms: Ancient Eastern Remedies for Modern Western Maladies," *Vegetarian Times* (March 1991): 64–68.

65. G. Chihara, "Medical Aspects of Lentinan Isolated from *Lentinus edodes* (Berk.) Sing," in *Mushroom Biology and Mushroom Products*, proceedings of the First International Conference on Mushroom Biology and Mushroom Products, Hong Kong, August 23–26, 1993, eds., Shu-ting Chang et al. (Shatin, Hong Kong: Chinese University Press, 1993), 261–66.

66. T. Nishizawa et al., "Homeostasis As Regulated by Activated Macrophage. I. Lipopolysaccharide (LPS) from Wheat Flour: Isolation, Purification and Some Biological Activities," *Chemical and Pharmaceutical Bulletin* 40 (1992): 479–83.

67. H. Inagawa et al., "Homeostasis As Regulated by Activated Mactrophage. II. LPS of Plant Origin Other Than Wheat Flour and Their Concomitant Bacteria," *Chemical and Pharmaceutical Bulletin* 40 (1992): 994–97.

68. G. Chihara, "Immunopharmacology of Lentinan, a Polysaccharide Isolated from *Lentinus edodes*: Its Application As a Host Defense Potentiator," *International Journal of Oriental Medicine* 17 (1992): 57–77.

CHAPTER FIVE

1. C. Servas, "Dr. Vincent Devita Speaks Out on Cancer Prevention with Fiber," *Saturday Evening Post* (August 1984): 51–56.

2. S. Findlay, "New Diet Guidelines to Prevent Cancer," *USA Today*, weekend edition, February 10–12, 1984.

3. M. Malkovsky et al., "Enhancement of Specific Antitumor Immunity in Mice Fed a Diet Enriched in Vitamin A Acetate," *Proceedings of the National Academy of Sciences USA* 80 (1983): 6322–26.

4. H. Padh, "Vitamin C: Newer Insights into Its Biochemical Functions," *Nutrition Reviews* 49 (March 1991): 65–70.

5. L. W. Wattenberg, "Chemoprevention of Cancer," *Cancer Research* 45 (1985): 1–8.

6. L. W. Wattenberg et al., "Inhibitory Effects of Phenolic Compounds on Benzo (2) Pyrene-Induced Neoplasias," *Cancer Research* 40 (1980): 2820–23.

7. L. W. Wattenberg et al., "Induction of Increased Benzopyrene Hydroxylase Activity by Flavones and Related Compounds," *Cancer Research* 28 (1968): 934–37.

8. W. Albert-Puleo, "Physiological Effects of Cabbage with Reference to Its Potential As a Dietary Cancer-Inhibitor and Its Use in Ancient Medicine," *Journal of Ethnopharmacology* 9 (1983): 261–72.

9. D. Pearson and S. Shaw, *Life Extension* (New York: Warner Books, 1982), 31, 261, 339, 410.

10. P. K. Ray et al., "Immunological Responses to Aflatoxins and Other Chemical Carcinogens," *Journal of Toxicology-Nutrition Reviews* 10 (1991): 63–85.

11. T. Knight et al., "Estimation of Dietary Intake of Nitrate and Nitrite in Great Britain," *Food Chemistry and Toxicology* 25 (1987): 277–85.

12. M. Nagao et al., "Nitrosatable Precursors of Mutagens in Vegetables and Soy Sauce," in *Diet, Nutrition and Cancer*, eds., Y. Hayashi et al. (Tokyo: Japan Science Society Press, 1986), 77–86. See also, G.-I. Danno et al., *Journal of Agriculture and Food Chemistry* 41 (1993): 1090–93.

13. See note 11 above.

14. D. A. Wagner et al., "Effect of Vitamin C and E on Endogenous Synthesis of *N*-Nitrosamino Acids in Humans: Precursor Product Studies with [^{15}N]Nitrate," *Cancer Research* 45 (1985): 6519–22.

15. S.-H. Lu et al., "Urinary Excretion of *N*-Nitrosamino Acids and Nitrate by Inhabitants of High- and Low-Risk Areas for Esophageal Cancer in Northern China: Endogenous Formation of Nitrosoproline and Its Inhibition by Vitamin C," *Cancer Research* 46 (1986): 1485–91.

16. S. E. Shephard et al., "Assessment of the Risk of Formation of Carcinogenic *N*-Nitroso Compounds from Dietary Precursors in the Stomach," *Food and Chemical Technology* 25 (1987): 91–108.

17. S. R. Tannenbaum et al., "The Effect of Nitrate Intake on Nitrite Formation in Human Saliva," *Food and Cosmetics Toxicology* 14 (1976): 549–52.

18. See note 12 above.

19. See note 11 above.

20. D. J. Stuehr and M. A. Marletta, "Mammalian Nitrate Biosynthesis: Mouse Macrophages Produce Nitrite and Nitrate in Response to *Escherichia coli* Lipopolysaccharide," *Proceedings of the National Academy of Sciences USA* 82 (1985): 7738–42.

21. J. B. Hibbs et al., "Macrophage Cytotoxicity: Role for *L*-Arginine Deiminase and Imino Nitrogen Oxidation to Nitrite," *Science* 235 (1987): 473–76.

22. W. E. W. Roediger et al., "Nitrite from Inflammatory Cells—A Cancer Risk Factor in Ulcerative Colitis?" *Diseases of the Colon and Rectum* 33 (1990): 1034–36.

23. Y. Kurashima et al., "Marked Formation of Thiazolidine-4-Carboxylic Acid, An Effective Nitrite Trapping Agent *in Vivo*, on Boiling of Dried Shiitake Mushroom (*Lentinus edodes*)," *Journal of Agriculture and Food Chemistry* 38 (1990): 1945–49.

24. F. Bollier and M. Martin, "L'Acido Tiazolidin-Carbossilico in Epatologia," *Gazzetta Medica Italiana* 131 (1972): 251–55 (in Italian).

25. A. Balsamo et al., "Is the Conformation of the Thiazolidine Ring of Penicillins of Any Importance for Their Antibacterial Activity? *European Journal of Medicinal Chemistry* 15 (1980): 559–62.

26. H. U. Weber et al., "Thiazolidine-4-Carboxylic Acid, a Physiologic Sulfhydryl Antioxidant with Potential Value in Geriatric Medicine," *Archives of Gerontology and Geriatrics* 1 (1982): 299–310.

27. See note 23 above.

28. T. Tahira et al., "The Inhibitory Effect of Thioproline on Carcinogenesis Induced by *N*-Benzylmethylamine and Nitrite," *Food Chemistry and Toxicology* 26 (1988): 511–16.

29. See note 26 above.

30. R. Bartoc et al., "Effect of Age and -SH Active Groups on the Activity of Some Enzymes Involved in the Carbohydrate Metabolism," *Experimental Gerontology* 10 (1975): 161–64.

31. See note 26 above.

32. G. Giorgi et al., "L-2-Oxothiazolidine-4-Carboxylic Acid and Glutathione in Human Immunodeficiency Virus Infection," *Current Therapeutic Research* 52 (1992): 461–67.

33. See note 23 above.

34. Ibid.

35. M. Tsuda et al., "Marked Increase in the Urinary Level of *N*-Nitrosothioproline after Ingestion of Cod with Vegetables," *Cancer Research* 48 (1988): 4049–52. See also note 23 above.

36. E. D. Gorham et al., "Sunlight and Breast Cancer Incidence in the USSR," *International Journal of Epidemiology* 19 (1990): 820–24.

37. C. Garland et al., "Dietary Vitamin D and Calcium and Risk of Colorectal Cancer: A 19-Year Prospective Study in Men," *The Lancet* 1 (1985): 307–9.

38. C. F. Garland et al., "Serum 25-Hydroxyvitamin D and Colon Cancer: Eight-Year Prospective Study," *The Lancet* 2 (1989): 1176–78.

39. C. F. Garland et al., "Geographic Variation in Breast Cancer Mortality in the United States: A Hypothesis Involving Exposure to Solar Radiation," *Preventive Medicine* 19 (1990): 614–22.

40. G. Cowley, "Can Sunshine Save Your Life? Vitamin D May Help Fight Colon and Breast Cancer," *Newsweek,* December 30, 1991, 56.

41. K. W. Colston et al., "Possible Role for Vitamin D in Controlling Breast Cancer Cell Proliferation," *The Lancet* 1 (January 28, 1989): 188–91.

42. B. C. Pence and F. Buddingh, "Inhibition of Dietary Fat-Promoted Colon Carcinogenesis in Rats by Supplemental Calcium or Vitamin D," *Carcinogenesis* 9 (1988): 187–90.

43. J. Teas, "The Dietary Intake of Laminaria, a Brown Seaweed, and Breast Cancer Prevention," *Nutrition and Cancer* 4 (1983): 217–22. See also note 40 above.

44. See note 36 above.

45. See note 38 above.

46. See note 39 above.

47. Ibid.

48. See note 40 above.

49. X.-P. Yu et al., "Vitamin D Receptor Expression in Human Lymphocytes," *Journal of Biological Chemistry* 266 (1991): 7588–95.

50. I. Serano et al., "*In Vitro* Effect of 1,25-Dihydroxyvitamin D3 (1,25–OH2D3) on NK Cell Cytotoxicity," in *Vitamin D*, proceedings of the Eighth Workshop on Vitamin D, Paris, France, July 5–10, 1991, eds., A. W. Norman et al. (New York: Walter de Gruyter, 1991), 496–97.

51. P. Sansoni et al., "1.25(OH)2D3 Increases Natural Killer (NK) Cell Activity," in *Vitamin D*, proceedings of the Eighth Workshop on Vitamin D, Paris, France,

July 5–10, 1991, eds., A. W. Norman et al. (New York: Walter de Gruyter, 1991), 512–13.

52. L. Rauova et al., "The *In Vivo* Effect of Vitamin D on Lymphocyte Subsets," in *Vitamin D*, proceedings of the Eighth Workshop on Vitamin D, Paris, France, July 5–10, 1991, eds., A. W. Norman et al. (New York: Walter de Gruyter, 1991), 508–9.

53. T. Kobayashi et al., "Shiitake and Vitamin D," *Vitamin* 62 (1988): 483–90 (in Japanese), in *Chemical Abstracts* 109 (1988): 23 (C.A.109:209885f).

54. J. Timmer et al., "A Nutritional Analysis and Development of Promotional Materials for Shiitake Mushroom Producers in Wisconsin," *Shiitake News* 7, no. 3 (1990): 6–11.

55. See note 40 above.

56. K. Mori, *Mushrooms As Health Foods* (Tokyo: Japan Publications, 1974), 29.

57. Ibid., 60.

58. A. H. Kryger, *Lentinan and the AIDS Epidemic*. Carmel, Calif., April 1985, unpublished, 6 pp.

59. C. Iizuka, "Antiviral Substance and the Manufacturing Method Thereof," *United States Patent* 4,629,627, December 16, 1986.

60. K. Mori et al., "Antitumor Activities of Edible Mushrooms by Oral Administration," in *Cultivating Edible Fungi*, International Symposium on Scientific and Technical Aspects of Cultivating Edible Fungi (IMS '86), Pennsylvania State University, July 15–17, 1986. Proceedings, eds., P. J. Wuest et al. (Elsevier, 1987), 1–6.

61. Ibid.

62. Ibid.

63. H. Nanba et al., "Antitumor Action of Shiitake (*Lentinus edodes*) Fruit Bodies Orally Administered to Mice," *Chemical and Pharmaceutical Bulletin* 35 (1987): 2453–58.

64. H. Nanba and H. Huroda, "Antitumor Mechanisms of Orally Administered Shiitake Fruit Bodies," *Chemical and Pharmaceutical Bulletin* 35 (1987): 2459–64.

65. See note 63 above.

66. See note 64 above.

67. Ibid.

68. N. Sugano et al., "Anticarcinogenic Action of an Alcohol-Insoluble Fraction (LAP1) from Culture Medium of *Lentinus edodes* Mycelia," *Cancer Letters* 27 (1985): 1–6.

69. Y. Suzuki et al., "Antitumor Effect of Water-Soluble Fraction Prepared from Culture Medium of *Lentinus edodes* Mycelia on Colonic Tumors Induced by Azoxymethane in Rats," *Journal of the Japanese Society of Colo-Proctology* 43 (1990): 177–91.

70. T. Suzuki and T. Ikegawa, "Anticancer Substance, Emitanin," in *Chemical Abstracts* 87 (1977): 539 (C.A. 199155d).

71. T. Suzuki and T. Ikegawa, "Method to Manufacture Anticancer Substance," *Japanese Patent* 77 79,087, December 25, 1975. 8 pp. Translated.

72. N. Sugano et al., "Anticarcinogenic Actions of Water-Soluble and Alcohol-Insoluble Fractions from Culture Medium of *Lentinus edodes* Mycelia," *Cancer Letters* 17 (1982): 109–14. See also notes 68 and 69 above.

73. T. Fujii et al., "Isolation and Characterization of a New Antitumor Polysaccharide, KS-2, Extracted from Culture Mycelia of *Lentinus edodes*," *Journal of Antibiotics* 31 (1978): 1079–90.

74. Ibid.

75. N. Ishida et al., "Antitumor Agent KS-2-B," *European Patent Application* 2 023 131, December 28, 1979.

76. See note 58 above.

77. A. H. Kryger, *The Lentinan Phenomenon,* Carmel, Calif., October 1983, unpublished. 4 pp.

78. See note 58 above.

79. See note 77 above.

80. H. Hanaue et al., "Changes in Blood Lymphocyte Subsets by Oral Administration of BRM," *Digestive Organ and Immunology,* no. 20 (1988): 78–82 (in Japanese), in *Chemical Abstracts* 110: 69099w.

81. H. Hanaue et al., "Effects of Oral Lentinan on T-Cell Subsets in Peripheral Venous Blood," *Clinical Therapeutics* 11 (1989): 614–22.

82. F. Levi et al., "Chronoimmunomodulation: Circadian, Circaseptan and Circannual Aspects of Immunopotentiation or Suppression with Lentinan," in *Toward Chronopharmacology*, Symposium: Eighth International Congress of Pharmacology, Nagasaki, Japan, July 27–28, 1981, ed., R. Takahashi (New York: Pergamon Press, 1982), 289–311.

83. U. Suzuki et al., "Abrogation of Oral Tolerance by Contrasuppressor T Cells Suggests the Presence of Regulatory T-Cell Networks in the Mucosal Immune System," *Nature* 320 (April 3, 1986): 451–54.

84. "Beta Carotene and the Immune System," in *Treatment Update,* no. 24 (June 1991): 5.

CHAPTER SIX

1. H. Miyakoshi et al., "Antigens of HTLV-I/or-III and Their Antibodies As Clinical Criteria for the Efficacy of Lentinan Administration," *International Journal of Immunopharmacology* 7 (1985): 331.

2. T. Aoki et al., "Antibodies to HTLV-I and III in Sera from Two Japanese Patients, One with Possible Pre-AIDS," *The Lancet* (October 20, 1984): 936–37.

3. J. S. James, "Suppressor Cells and Alternative AIDS/ARC Treatments," *AIDS Treatment News,* no. 20 (December 19, 1986): 2–3.

4. L. Badgley, *Healing AIDS Naturally* (West San Bruno, Calif.: Human Energy Press, 1988). See also note 1 above.

5. See note 2 above.

6. R. C. Gallo, "My Life Stalking AIDS," *Discover* magazine, October 1989, 31–36.

7. V. Zaninovic et al., "Origins of T-Cell Leukemia Virus," *Nature* 344 (March 22, 1990): 299.

8. G. Cowley, "The Future of AIDS," *Newsweek*, March 22, 1993, 46–52.

9. Ibid.

10. P. W. Ewald, "The Evolution of Virulence," *Scientific American,* April 1993, 86–93.

11. M. Mochizuki et al., "HTLV-I Uveitis: A Distinct Clinical Entity Caused by HTLV-I," *Japanese Journal of Cancer Research* 83 (1992): 236–39.

12. P. A. Bunn et al., "Clinical Course of Retrovirus-Associated Adult T-Cell Lymphoma in the United States," *New England Journal of Medicine* 309 (August 4, 1983): 257–64.

13. P. M. S. de Oliveira et al., "Adult T-Cell Leukemia/Lymphoma in Brazil and Its Relation to HTLV-I," *The Lancet* 336 (October 20, 1990): 987–89.

14. See note 7 above.

15. See note 2 above.

16. Ibid.

17. J. S. James, "AZT, Alternatives, and Public Policy," *AIDS Treatment News,* no. 28 (March 27, 1987): 4.

18. See note 3 above.

19. See note 2 above.

20. K. Graven, "Japanese Join World Push to Cure AIDS," *Wall Street Journal*, November 10, 1988, B4.

21. J. Matsuda et al., "Amelioration of Deteriorated Polymorphonuclear Leukocyte (PMN) Phagocytic Function of Hemophiliacs with HIV Infection by Administration of Long-Term Polysaccharide Immunopotentiator (Lentinan)," in *Fifth International Conference on AIDS*, Abstracts, Montreal, Quebec, Canada, June 4–9, 1989. International Development Research Centre, Ottawa, Ontario, 1989: 403.

22. J. S. James, "San Francisco: Lentinan Study Recruiting," *AIDS Treatment News,* no. 73 (January 27, 1989): 5.

23. G. Dennert and D. Tucker, "Antitumor Polysaccharide Lentinan—A T Cell Adjuvant," *Journal of the National Cancer Institute* 18 (1976): 93–104.

24. S. Hara et al., "Selective Suppression of T-Cell Activity in Tumor-Bearing Mice and Its Improvement by Lentinan, a Potent Antitumor Polysaccharide," *International Journal of Cancer* 18 (1976): 93–104.

25. A. H. Kryger, *The Lentinan Phenomenon,* Carmel, Calif., October 1983, unpublished. 4 pp.

26. T. Aoki, "Lentinan," in *Immune Modulating Agents and Their Mechanisms,* eds., R. L. Fenishel and M. A. Chirgis (New York and Basel: Marcel Dekker, 1984), 63–77.

27. Y. Kaneko et al., "Activity of Lentinan Against Cancer and AIDS," *International Journal of Immunotherapy* 5 (1989): 203–13.

28. Personal communication of Maxwell Gordon, Lentico-Chemico Pharmaceutical Laboratory, October 8, 1991.

29. "Lentinan," in *AIDS/HIV Treatment Directory* 4, no. 4 (April 1991): 24.

30. D. Abrams et al., "Results of a Phase I/II Placebo-Controlled Dose Finding Pilot Study of Lentinan in Patients with HIV Infection," in *Sixth International Conference on AIDS,* vol. 3, abstracts. University of California, San Francisco, June 20–24, 1990, 207: abstr. S.B. 487.

31. L. Meyaard et al., "T Cell Dysfunction in HIV Infection: Anergy Due to Defective Antigen-Presenting Cell Function," *Immunology Today* 14, no. 4 (1993): 161–64.

32. M. R. Helbert et al., "Antigen Presentation, Loss of Immunological Memory and AIDS," *Immunology Today* 14, no. 7 (1993): 340–43.

33. H. S. L. M. Nottet et al., "Down-Regulation of Human Immunodeficiency Virus Type 1 (HIV-1) Production after Stimulation of Monocyte-Derived Macrophages Infected with HIV-1," *Journal of Infectious Diseases* 167 (1993): 810–17.

34. T. S. Tochikura et al., "Suppression of Human Immunodeficiency Virus Replication by 3'-Azido-3'-Deoxythymidine in Various Human Hematopoeic Cell Lines *in Vitro:* Augmentation of the Effect by Lentinan," *Japanese Journal of Cancer Research* 78 (1987): 583–89. See also note 27 above.

35. See note 27 above.

36. See note 28 above.

37. "ddI," in *AIDS/HIV Treatment Directory* 4, no. 4 (April 1991): 13–15.

38. G. Torres, "AZT/ddI Highlights from European AIDS Conference," *TreatmentIssues* 6, no. 5 (1992): 1–2.

39. G. Torres, "VII International Conference on AIDS: Antiretroviral Update," *Treatment Issues* 6, no. 8 (1992): 1–2.

40. P. Cotton, "Immune Boosters Disappoint AIDS Researchers," *Journal of the American Medical Association* 266 (September 25, 1991): 1613–14.

41. *The Journal: Have a Talk with Owners* 129 (January 1982): 18–23 (Tokyo monthly magazine in Japanese, translated).

42. H. Yahara, *Shukan Gendai (Weekly Magazine Today),* December 17, 1983, 219–22 (Tokyo weekly magazine, translated).

43. Y. Sugi, *Seijikai* (*Political World*) 20 (September 1981): 66–68 (Tokyo monthly magazine, translated).

44. C. Iizuka, "Antiviral Substance and the Manufacturing Method Thereof," *United States Patent* 4,629,627, December 16, 1986. See also H. Amagase, "Treatment of Hepatitis B Patients with *Lentinus edodes* Mycelium," *Excerpta Medica*, 1987, 316–21. Amagase's research was a pilot study. It was conducted without a placebo control group and would have to be repeated to learn the real success rate of LEM against hepatits B.

45. See notes 41 to 44 above.

46. See note 44 above.

47. S. Tochikura et al., "Inhibition (*in Vitro*) of Replication and of the Cytopathic Effect of Human Immunodeficiency Virus by an Extract of the Culture Medium of *Lentinus edodes* Mycelia," *Medical Microbiology and Immunology 26* (1988): 1229–32.

48. N. Nakashima et al., "Rapid Screening Method with a Cell Multisizer for Inhibitors of Human Immunodeficiency Virus-Induced Cell Fusion *in Vitro*," *Journal of Clinical Microbiology* 26 (1988): 1229–32.

49. H. Suzuki et al., "Immunopotentiating Substances in *Lentinus edodes* Mycelial Extract (LEM)—Activation of Macrophages and Proliferation of Bone Marrow Cell," *Japanese Journal of Gastroenterology* 85 (1988): 1430.

50. I. L. Weismann and W. D. Cooper, "How the Immune System Develops," *Scientific American*, September 1993, 65–71.

51. H. Suzuki et al., "Inhibition of the Infectivity and Cytopathic Effect of Human Immunodeficiency Virus by Water-Soluble Lignin in an Extract of the Culture Medium of *Lentinus edodes* Mycelia (LEM)," *Biochemical and Biological Research Communications* 160 (1989): 367–73.

52. H. Suzuki et al., "Structural Characterization of the Immunoactive and Antiviral Water-Solubilized Lignin in an Extract of the Culture Medium of *Lentinus edodes* Mycelia (LEM)," *Agricultural and Biological Chemistry* 54 (1990): 479–87.

53. See note 51 above.

54. Ibid.

55. K. Sorimachi et al., "Antiviral Activity of Water-Solubilized Lignin Derivatives *in Vitro*," *Agricultural and Biological Chemistry* 54 (1990): 1337–39.

56. F. Hanafusa et al., "Intestinal Absorption and Tissue Distribution of Immunoactive and Antiviral Water-Soluble [^{16}C] Lignins in Rats," *Yakubutsu Dotai* 5 (1990): 661–74 (in Japanese), in *Chemical Abstracts* 114 (1991): 13–14 (C.A. 114: 220685q).

57. K. Yamafuji and H. Murakami, "Antitumor Potency of Lignin and Pyrocatechol and Their Action on Deoxyribonucleic Acid," *Enzymologia* 35 (1968): 139–53.

58. C. Iizuka, "Therapeutic Agent for AIDS," *European Patent Application*, EP 0 370 673 A3, June 27, 1990.

59. See notes 44 and 51 above.

60. C. Iizuka et al., "Manufacture of Antiviral Glycoprotein with Basidiomycete," *Japanese Patent* 02,286,623, November 26, 1990, *Chemical Abstracts* 114 (1991): 616 (C.A. 114: 162433t).

61. See note 58 above.

62. A. Shirahata et al., "The Usefulness of LEM (the Extract of Cultured Lentinus edodes Mycelia) in HIV-Infected Hemophiliacs," in *Sixth International Conference on AIDS*, vol. 2., abstracts. University of California, San Francisco, June 20–24, 1990, 372: abstr. 2074. See also note 58 above.

63. Ibid.

64. N. Sugano et al., "Immunopotentiation Agents," *European Patent Application* EP 154 066, September 11, 1985.

65. T. Sharon, Information Summary: *Lentinus edodes (Shiitake) Mycelial Extract*. LEM Survey Project, El Torro, Calif., March 13, 1989. 10 pp.

66. See notes 58 and 62 above.

67. Dr. K. L. Jones, press release, "Herpes, Allergy and AIDS Patients Improve," Westwood, California, July 27, 1985.

68. Dr. Mosleh, "Test Data Regarding the Use of C-Kin, A Shiitake Mycelial Extract," Emperor's College of Traditional Oriental Medicine, July 27, 1985. See also note 62 above.

69. See notes 67 and 68 above.

70. Ibid.

71. Dr. K. L. Jones, AIDS *Experimental Protocol*, Westwood, California, undated.

72. "NIH Studies Lymph Nodes," *TreatmentUpdate* 4, no. 4 (1993): 3.

73. See note 33 above.

74. H. M. Temin and D. P. Bolognesi, "Where Has HIV Been Hiding?" *Nature* 362 (1993): 292–93.

75. G. Pantelo et al., "HIV Infection Is Active and Progressive in Lymphoid Tissue During the Clinically Latent Stage of Disease," *Nature* 362 (1993): 353–58.

76. J. Embretson et al., "Massive Covert Infection of Helper T Lymphocytes and Macrophages by HIV During the Incubation Period of AIDS," *Nature* 362 (1993): 359–62.

77. S. Straus, "HIV Hides in Glands, Scientists Discover: Earlier Treatment of AIDS Possible," *Globe and Mail*, Toronto, March 25, 1993, A1 and A2.

78. G. Cowley with M. Hagar, "Sleeping with the Enemy," *Newsweek*, December 9, 1991, 58–59.

79. R. Stein, "The ABC's of Hepatitis: The Viruses That Cause Liver Disease Grow Ever More Insidious," *American Health*, June 1993, 65–69.

80. Ibid.

81. "High Rate of Hepatitis, HIV Found in City Hospital ERs," *American Pharmacy* NS32, no. 8 (August 1992): 12.

82. "Efforts Intensify to Curb Hepatitis B," *American Pharmacy* NS32, no. 8 (August 1992): 12.

83. Y. Ghendon, "WHO Strategy for the Global Elimination of New Cases of Hepatitis B," *Vaccine* 8, suppl. (1990): S129–S133.

84. See note 79 above.

85. M. I. Thabrew et al., "Immunomodulatory Activity of Three Sri-Lankan Medicinal Plants Used in Hepatic Disorders," *Journal of Ethnopharmacology* 33 (1991): 63–6.

86. See note 44 above.

87. See note 67 above.

88. See note 44 above.

89. Y. Mizoguchi et al., "Effects of Extract of Cultured *Lentinus edodes* Mycelia (LEM) on Polyclonal Antibody Responses Induced by Pokeweed Mitogen," *Gastroenterologia Japonica* 22 (1987): 627–32.

90. Y. Mizoguchi et al., "Protection of Liver Cells Against Experimental Damage by Extract of Cultured *Lentinus edodes* Mycelia (LEM)," *Gastroenterologia Japonica* 22 (1987): 459–64.

91. J. D. Mosca, "Herpes and AIDS," in *Cofactors in HIV-1 Infection and AIDS*, ed., R. R. Watson (Boca Raton, Fla.: CRC Press, 1989), 201–16.

92. See note 44 above.

93. Ibid.

94. J. Koga et al., "Anti-Viral Fraction of Aqueous Lentinus edodes Extract," *European Patent Application* EP 437 346 A1, July 17, 1991.

95. See note 68 above.

96. Ibid.

97. Ibid.

98. See note 67 above.

99. Ibid.

100. American Immunological Society, letter to the editor, *Townsend Letter for Doctors,* no. 117 (April 1993): 325–27. See also note 78 above.

101. K. Helsen and G. R. Kinghorn, "Extragenital Complication of Genital Herpes," *British Journal of Sexual Medicine* 18 (1991): 8–11.

CHAPTER SEVEN

1. T. Aoki et al., "Administration of Lentinan to Patients with Immune Depression Disease (IDD)," *International Journal of Immunopharmacology* 7 (1985): 331.

2. T. Aoki et al., "Low Natural Killer Syndrome: Clinical and Immunological Features," *Natural Immunity and Cell Growth Regulation* 6 (1987): 116–28.

3. M. Caliguri et al., "Phenotypic and Functional Deficiency of Natural Killer Cells in Patients with Chronic Fatigue Syndrome," *Journal of Immunology* 139 (1987): 3306–13.

4. N. Ostrom, "LEM: Is It the Vitamin C of the Immune System?" *CFIDS Chronicle* (Summer/Fall 1989): 44–47.

5. See note 1 above.

6. See note 2 above.

7. Ibid.

8. T. Aoki et al., "Antibodies to HTLV I and III in Sera from Two Japanese Patients, One with Possible Pre-AIDS," *The Lancet* (October 20, 1984): 936–37.

9. T. Aoki, "Lentinan," in *Immune Modulation Agents and Their Mechanisms*, eds., R. L. Fenishel and M. A. Chirgis (New York and Basel: Marcel Dekker, 1984), 63–77.

10. Ibid.

11. Ibid.

12. J. S. James, "Shiitake, Lentinan, and AIDS," *AIDS Treatment News,* December 5, 1986.

13. G. Chihara et al., "Fractionation and Purification of the Polysaccharides with Marked Antitumor Activity, Especially Lentinan, from *Lentinus edodes* (Berk.) Sing. (An Edible Mushroom)," *Cancer Research* 30 (1970): 2776–81.

14. H. Namba et al., "Antitumor Action of Shiitake (*Lentinus edodes*) Fruit Bodies Orally Administered to Mice," *Chemical and Pharmaceutical Bulletin* 35 (1987): 2453–58. See also note 13 above.

15. N. L. Eby et al., "Natural Killer Cell Activity in the Chronic Fatigue–Immune Dysfunction Syndrome," in *Natural Killer Cells and Host Defense*. Fifth International Natural Killer Cell Workshop, Hilton Head, South Carolina, 1988 (Basel: Karger, 1989), 141–45.

16. S. Grufferman, "Abnormalities in Immune System in Patients with Chronic Fatigue Syndrome," *The Nightingale* 1, no. 3 (1990): 12 (abstract).

17. M. Irwin and J. C. Gillin, "Impaired Natural Killer Cell Activity Among Depressed Patients," *Psychiatry Research* 20 (1987): 181–82.

18. M. Irwin, "Depression and Immune Function," *Stress Medicine* 14 (1988): 95–103.

19. M. Irwin et al., "Reduction of Immune Function in Life Stress and Depression," *Biological Psychiatry* 27 (1990): 22–30.

20. B. A. Cunha, "Beta-Carotene Stimulation of Natural Killer Cell Activity in Adult Patients with Chronic Fatigue Syndrome," *CFIDS Chronicle* (Fall 1993): 18–19.

21. E. Leyton and H. Pross, "Chronic Fatigue Syndrome: Do Herbs and Homeopathy Help?" *Canadian Family Physician* 38 (1992): 2021–26. See also note 3 above.

22. N. Ostram, "Why Peter Duesberg May Still Be Wrong About AIDS and Chronic Fatigue Syndrome," *New York Native,* March 18, 1991.

23. B. Hyde, "Myalgic Encephalomyelitis: The Name, Definition, and Classification," C*FIDS Chronicle* (Summer 1989): 37–40. See also E. A. Ojo-Amaize et al., "Decreased Natural Killer Cell Activity Is Associated with Severity of Chronic Fatigue Immune Dysfunction Syndrome," *Clinical Infectious Diseases* 18, suppl. 1 (1994): S157–59.

24. J. Reilly, "LEM: Suppressor of My Demon," *CFIDS Buyers Club Newsletter,* Santa Barbara, Calif., Fall 1991: 10–11.

25. Dr. C. A. Mildon, *The Saga of the Prolonged Viral Syndrome*, lecture handout, address to Ontario Claims Association, Peterborough, Ontario, January 14, 1988. 12 pp.

26. See notes 23, 24, and 25 above.

27. M. Sharpe et al., "Follow Up of Patients Presenting with Fatigue to an Infectious Diseases Clinic," *British Medical Journal* 305 (1992): 147–52.

28. R. E. Kendell, "Chronic Fatigue, Viruses, and Depression," *The Lancet* 337 (January 19, 1991): 160–62.

29. M. A. Demitrack et al., "Evidence for Impaired Activation of the Hypothalamic-Pituitary-Adrenal Axis in Patients with Chronic Fatigue Syndrome," *Journal of Clinical Endocrinology and Metabolism* 73 (1991): 1224–34.

30. P. R. Cheney et al., "The Diagnosis of Chronic Fatigue Syndrome: An Assertive Approach," *CFIDS Chronicle* (September 1992): 13–19.

31. Ibid.

32. M. Maes et al., "Evidence for a Systemic Immune Activation During Depression: Results of Leukocyte Enumeration by Flow Cytometry in Conjunction with Monoclonal Antibody Staining," *Psychological Medicine* 22 (1992): 45–53.

33. D. R. Denney et al., "Lymphocyte Subclasses and Depression," *Journal of Abnormal Psychology* 97 (1988): 499–502.

34. News Release, The CFIDS Association of America, Inc., Charlotte, N.C., February 8, 1993, "Government Finally Confirms Private Sector Research: Immune Abnormalities Found in Chronic Fatigue Syndrome."

35. News Release, National Institutes of Health, "Immune Abnormalities Found in Chronic Fatigue Syndrome May Lead to Better Understanding of the Disease," *Townsend Letter for Doctors,* no. 118 (May 1993): 504.

36. S. E. Straus et al., "Lymphocyte Phenotype and Function in the Chronic Fatigue Syndrome," *Journal of Clinical Immunology* 13 (1993): 30–40.

37. See note 32 above.

38. See notes 35 and 36 above.

39. C. Jessop, "Clinical Features and Possible Etiology of CFIDS," *CFIDS Chronicle* (Spring 1991): 70–73.

40. J. A. Goldstein, "The Diagnosis of Chronic Fatigue Syndrome As a Limbic Encephalopathy," *CFIDS Chronicle* (September 1992): 20–34.

41. See notes 35 and 36 above.

42. E. A. Bachen et al., "Lymphocyte Subset and Cellular Immune Responses to a Brief Experimental Stressor," *Psychosomatic Medicine* 54 (1992): 673–79.

43. M. Stein et al., "Stress and Immunostimulation: The Role of Depression and Neuroendocrine Function," *Journal of Immunology* 135 (1985): 827s–33s.

44. M. R. Irwin et al., "Adaptation to Chronic Stress. Temporal Pattern of Immune and Neuroendocrine Correlates," *Neuropsychopharmacology* 1 (1988): 239–42.

45. R. Glaser et al., "Stress Depresses Interferon Production by Leukocytes Concomitant with a Decrease in Natural Killer Cell Activity," *Behavioral Neuroscience* 100 (1986): 675–78.

46. Y. Kusaka et al., "Healthy Lifestyles are Associated with Higher Natural Killer Cell Activity," *Preventive Medicine* 21 (1992): 602–15.

47. Ibid.

48. Myron Brenton. *Help for the Troubled Employee,* Public Affairs Pamphlet No. 611 (New York: Public Affairs Committee, 1982), 3.

49. L. M. Iger, "The MMPI-2 Chronic Fatigue Syndrome Profile," *CFIDS Chronicle* (September 1992): 61–65.

50. *Chronic Fatigue Syndrome: A Pamphlet for Physicians,* U.S. Dept. of Health and Human Services, National Institutes of Health, NIH Publication No. 92–484, May 1992. 15 pp.

51. C. W. Lapp, "Chronic Fatigue Syndrome Is a *Real* Disease," *North Carolina Family Physician* 43 (1992): 6–11.

52. CDC CFS Research Group, Centers for Disease Control, Atlanta, Georgia, "Chronic Fatigue Syndrome Research at the Centers for Disease Control," *CFIDS Chronicle Physician's Forum* (September 1992): 50–52.

53. *How Many People Have CFIDS?* Handout, citing testimony of E. DeFreitas, Ph.D., of the Wistar Institute, before the U.S. House Subcommittee on Health and the Environment, April 16, 1991. The CFIDS Association, Inc., P.O. Box 220398, Charlotte, NC 28222–0398.

54. S. E. Straus, "The Chronic Mononucleosis Syndrome," *Journal of Infectious Diseases* 157 (1988): 405–12.

55. Dr. C. Shepherd, *Living with M.E.* (London: Cedar Books, 1989), 13–22.

56. J. Goldstein, "Presumed Pathogenesis and Treatment of the Chronic Fatigue Syndrome," *The Nightingale* 1, no. 3 (1990): 11 (abstract).

57. E. DeFreitas et al., "Retroviral Sequences Related to Human T-Lymphotropic Virus Type II in Patients with Chronic Fatigue Immune Dysfunction Syndrome," *Proceedings of the National Academy of Sciences USA* 88 (1991): 2922–26.

58. N. Ostram, "CIDS Retrovirus: Cause or Co-Factor," *New York Native*, April 15, 1991, 23.

59. D. R. Lucey, "The First Decade of Human Retroviruses: A Nomenclature for the Clinician," *Journal of Military Medicine* 156 (1991): 555–57.

60. P. Lusso et al., "Infection of Natural Killer Cells by Human Herpesvirus 6," *Nature* 362 (April 1, 1993): 458–62.

61. M. Luppi et al., "Three Cases of Human Herpesvirus-6 Latent Infection: Integration of Viral Genome in Peripheral Blood Mononuclear Cell DNA," *Journal of Medical Virology* 40 (1993): 44–52.

62. See note 60 above.

63. See note 61 above.

64. *Dorland's Illustrated Medical Dictionary*, 26th edition (Philadelphia: W. B. Saunders, 1981), 472.

65. H. Agut, "Puzzles Concerning the Pathogenicity of Human Herpesvirus 6," *New England Journal of Medicine* 329 (1993): 203–4.

66. K. Akashi et al., "Brief Report: Severe Infectious Mononucleosis-Like Syndrome and Primary Human Herpesvirus 6 Infection in an Adult," *New England Journal of Medicine* 329 (1993): 168–71.

67. See note 57 above.

68. M. Kaplan et al., "HTLV-I and HTLV-II Infection in HIV Infected Patients: Report of 45 Coinfected Patients," in *Sixth International Conference on AIDS, San Francisco, California, June 20–24, 1990, Program Abstracts*, vol. 2: abstract F.C.670, p. 248.

69. H. H. Lee et al., "HTLV-I and HTLV-II Infection in U.S. Blood Donors Is Associated with Different Risk Factors," in *Sixth International Conference on AIDS, San Francisco, California, June 20–24, Program Abstracts*, vol. 1: Abstract Th.A.302, p. 195.

70. See note 19 above.

71. J. Regennitter, letter to the author, November 1991. See also note 24 above.

72. J. Regennitter, letter to the author, December 2, 1991.

73. See note 24 above.

74. Dr. J. A. Goldstein, *Chronic Fatigue Syndrome: The Struggle for Health* (Beverly Hills, Calif.: Chronic Fatigue Syndrome Institute, 1990), 105–49.

75. *CFIDS Buyer's Club NewsLetter* 2 (Fall 1991): 9–11.

76. J. Avery, letter to the editor, *CFIDS Buyer's Club Health Watch Newsletter* 11, no. 2 (1992): 11.

77. See notes 4, 74, and 75 above.

78. N. Ostram, "Unsung Hero: Former Stockbroker Rich Carson, Disabled by CIDS, Raises Hundreds of Thousands of Dollars for Research," *New York Native*, October 29, 1990.

79. R. Winslow, "New Drug May Help Chronic Fatigue Sufferers," *Wall Street Journal*, October 2, 1991. See also D. A. Strayer et al., "A Controlled Clinical Trial with a Specifically Configured RNA Drug, Poly(I)•Poly(C$_{12}$U), in Chronic Fatigue Syndrome," *Clinical Infectious Diseases* 18, suppl. 1(1994): S88–95.

80. See note 9 above.

81. T. Suzuki and T. Ikegawa, "Anticancer Substance, Emitanin," in *Chemical Abstracts* 87 (1977): 539 (C.A. 199155d).

82. T. Sharon, *Information Summary: Lentinus edodes (Shiitake) Mycelial Extract*. LEM Survey Project, El Torro, Calif., March 13, 1989. 10 pp.

83. C. Iizuka, "Antiviral Substance and the Manufacturing Method Thereof," *United States Patent* 4,629,627, December 16, 1986.

84. F. Suzuki et al., "Antiviral and Interferon-Inducing Activities of a New Peptidomannan, KS-2, Extracted from Culture Mycelia of *Lentinus edodes*," *Journal of Antibiotics* 32 (1979): 1336–44.

85. T. Fujii et al., "Isolation and Characterization of a New Antitumor Polysaccharide, KS-2, Extracted from Culture Mycelia of *Lentinus edodes*," *Journal of Antibiotics* 31 (1978): 1079–90.

86. F. Suzuki et al., "Antitumor Activity of KS-2 and Interferon-Inducing Activity," *Proceedings of the 36th Annual Meeting of the Japanese Cancer Association*, Tokyo, Japan, October 1977: 79.

87. A. Yamashita et al., "Intestinal Absorption and Urinary Excretion of Antitumor Peptidomannan KS-2 after Oral Administration in Rats," *Immunopharmacology* 5 (1983): 209–20.

88. Kirin-Seagram Limited, Tokyo, "Chemotherapeutic Substances and Methods of Manufacturing Same," *U.K. Patent* 1 572 74, July 23, 1980.

89. M. Togami et al., "Studies on Basidiomycetes. I. Antitumor Polysaccharide from Bagasse Medium on Which Mycelia of *Lentinus edodes* (Berk.) Sing. Had Been Grown," *Chemical and Pharmaceutical Bulletin* 30 (1982): 1134–40.

90. N. Sugano et al., "Anticarcinogenic Actions of Water-Soluble Fractions from Culture Medium of *Lentinus edodes* Mycelia," *Cancer Letters* 17 (1982): 109–14.

91. N. Sugano et al., "Anticarcinogenic Action of an Alcohol-Insoluble Fraction (LAP 1) from Culture Medium of *Lentinus edodes* Mycelia," *Cancer Letters* 27 (1985): 1–5.

92. See note 85 above.

93. See note 84 above.

94. See note 85 above.

95. Dr. D. L. Peterson, "Proposed Study of Lentinus Edodes Mycelia on Chronic Fatigue Syndrome," Incline Village, Nevada, undated, unpublished. 2 pp.

96. Dr. D. S. Bell, "Protocol for the Use of LEM (Lentinus edodes mycelia) in Chronic Fatigue Syndrome," February 6, 1989, Lyndonville, New York, unpublished.

Dr. David Bell is featured in an article on CFS in *Newsweek*, November 12, 1990, 62–70; CFS was the cover story.

97. J. A. Goldstein, "Functional Brain Imaging in CFIDS," *CFIDS Chronicle* (Spring 1991): 101–3. See also Dr. J. A. Goldstein, *Chronic Fatigue Syndromes: The Limbic Hypothesis* (New York: Haworth Medical Press, 1993).

98. See note 74 above.

99. Personal communication of L. Nielson, national director, Myalgic Encephalomyelitis Support and Help Group (M.E.S.H.), Ottawa, Ontario, December 10, 1991.

100. I. M. Cox et al., "Red Blood Cell Magnesium and Chronic Fatigue Syndrome," *The Lancet* 337 (March 30, 1991): 757–60. See also P.R. Cheney et al., "Entero-Hepatic Resuscitation in Patients with Chronic Fatigue Syndrome: A Pyramid of Nutritional Therapy," *CFIDS Chronicle Physicians' Forum* (Fall 1993):1–3.

101. P. O. Behan et al., "Effect of High Doses of Essential Fatty Acids on the Postviral Fatigue Syndrome," *Acta Neurologica Scandinavia* 82 (1990): 209–16.

102. P. O. Behan and W. M. H. Behan, "Essential Fatty Acids in the Treatment of Postviral Fatigue Syndrome," in *Omega-6 Essential Fatty Acids: Pathophysiology and Roles in Clinical Medicine*, ed., D. F. Horrobin (New York: Alan R. Liss, 1990), 275–82. Note that one study (double-blind, randomized, and placebo-controlled), lasting six months with a preparation of 80 percent evening primrose oil and 20 percent fish oil in ninety-eight CFS patients, failed to find any benefits. See S. J. McBride and D. R. McClusky, *British Medical Bulletin* 47 (1991): 895–907.

103. K. Kenney, "Ampligen: Past, Present and Future," *CFIDS Chronicle* 1, no. 1 (March 1991): 18–20. See also note 79 above.

104. T. L. Steinbach and W. J. Hermann, "The Treatment of CFIDS with Kutapressin™," *CFIDS Chronicle* (Spring/Summer 1990): 25–28. See also E. J. Conley, "Treatment of HHV-6 Reactivation in CFIDS," *CFIDS Chronicle Physicians' Forum* (Fall 1993): 15–17.

105. See notes 1 and 2 above.

106. "Anti-Cancer Mushroom Agent Shows Anti-CFS Activity," *Japan Economic Journal*, May 1, 1992, cited by Neenyah Ostram in "Another Mushroom Miracle," *New York Native*, June 29, 1992, 1–3.

107. H. S. Sklar et al., "CFS: Treatment with Adenosine Monophosphate," *CFIDS Chronicle* (Spring/Summer 1990): 170–71.

108. H. S. Sklar, "Study of AMP Treatment in CFIDS," *CFIDS Chronicle* (Spring 1989): 144.

109. M. M. Iverson, "Enter, Dr. Hyde," *CFIDS Chronicle* (Summer/Fall 1989): 35–36.

110. S. Jacobsen et al., "Oral S-Adenosylmethionine in Primary Fibromyalgia. Double-Blind Clinical Evaluation," *Scandinavian Journal of Rheumatology* 20 (1991): 294–302.

111. N. Komatsu et al., "Host-Mediated Antitumor Action of Schizophyllan, a Glucan Produced by *Schizophyllum commune*," *Japanese Journal of Cancer Research* 60 (1969): 137–44.

112. G. H. Lincoff, *The Audubon Society Field Guide to North American Mushrooms* (New York: Alfred A. Knopf, Chanticleer Press, 1981), 487, 493.

113. G. Parent and D. Thoen, "Food Value of Edible Mushrooms from Upper-Shaba Region," *Economic Botany* 31 (1977): 436–45.

114. M. A. M. Alfaro et al., "Etnomicología y Exploraciones Micologicas en la Sierra Norte de Puebla," *Boletím Sociedad Mexícana de Micologia* 18 (1983):51–63.

115. J. Ying et al., *Icones of Medicinal Fungi from China* (Beijing: Science Press, 1987), 283.

116. Q. Y. Yang and S. C. Jong, "Medicinal Mushrooms in China," in *Mushroom Science VII* (Part I), proceedings of the Twelfth International Congress on the Science and Cultivation of Edible Fungi, Braunschweig, Germany, 1987, eds., K. Grabbe and O. Hilber (Braunschweig, Germany: Institute for Bodenbiologie, 1989), 631–43.

117. N. Komatsu, "Biological Activities of Schizophyllan," in *Mushroom Science IX* (Part I), proceedings of the Ninth International Scientific Congress on the Cultivation of Edible Fungi, Tokyo, 1974 (Kiryu, Japan: Mushroom Research Institute, 1976), 867–70. See also note 110 above.

118. H. Furue, "Clinical Evaluation of Schizophyllan (SPG) in Gastric Cancer—Randomized Controlled Studies," in Abstracts of the Third International Conference on Immunopharmacology, May 6–9, 1985, Florence, Italy. *International Journal of Immunopharmacology* 7 (1985): 333.

119. K. Okamura et al., "Clinical Evaluation of Schizophyllan Combined with Irradiation on Patients with Cervical Cancer—A Randomized Controlled Study," in Abstracts of the Third International Conference on Immunopharmacology, May 6–9, 1985, Florence, Italy. *International Journal of Immunopharmacology* 7 (1985): 333.

120. K. Okamura et al., "Adjuvant Immunotherapy: Two Randomized Controlled Studies of Patients with Cervical Cancer," *Biomedicine and Pharmacotherapy* 43 (1989): 177–81.

121. I. Gorai et al., "Immunological Modulation of Lymphocyte Subpopulation in Cervical Cancer Tissue by Sizofiran and OK-432," *Gynecologic Oncology* 44 (1992): 137–46.

122. Y. Shimizu et al., "Augmenting Effect of Sizofiran on the Immunofunction of Regional Lymph Nodes in Cervical Cancer," *Cancer* 69 (1992): 1188–94.

123. K. Noda et al., "Clinical Effect of Sizofiran Combined with Irradiation in Cervical Cancer Patients: A Randomized Controlled Study," *Japanese Journal of Clinical Oncology* 22 (1992): 17–25.

124. See note 106 above.

125. Dr. A. Uchida, letter to the author, June 18, 1993.

126. A. Uchida et al., "Treatment with Sizofiran of Patients with Chronic Fatigue Syndrome: Restoration of Blood NK Cell Activity and Improvement of Clinical Symptoms," *Proceedings of the International Congress on Chemotherapy*. Publication pending.

127. See note 32 above.

128. See note 126 above.

129. Ibid.

130. See note 32 above.

131. M. Suzuki et al., "Induction of Endogenous Lymphokine-Activated Killer Activity by Combined Administration of Lentinan and Interleukin 2," *International Journal of Immunopharmacology* 12 (1990): 613–23.

132. A. J. Ramsay et al., "A Case for Cytokines As Effector Molecules in the Resolution of Virus Infection," *Immunology Today* 14 (1993): 155–57.

133. "TB Drugs: Clinical Trials and Drug Availability," *Treatment Issues* 10, no. 7 (1993): 2.

134. See note 126 above.

135. Ibid.

136. B. Hyde, "The Enterovirus Cause of M.E.," *CFIDS Chronicle* (Summer/Fall 1989): 155–58. See also note 99 above.

137. Ibid.

138. Ibid.

139. C. W. Lapp, "The Practical Treatment of CFIDS: One Doctor's Approach," *CFIDS Chronicle* (Summer/Fall 1989): 16–21.

140. K. Jones, "The *Oketsu* Syndrome and CFS," *Townsend Letter for Doctors,* no. 120 (July 1993): 688–93.

141. K. Mori, *Mushrooms As Health Foods* (Tokyo: Japan Publications, 1974), 29, 64–72.

142. A. L. Komaroff, "Chronic Fatigue Syndromes: Relationship to Chronic Viral Infections," *Journal of Virological Methods* 21 (1988): 3–10. See also notes 19, 39, and 40 above.

143. Editorial, "A British Definition of M.E.," *M.E. Association of Canada Newsletter* 1, no. 1 (January/February 1989): 5–7.

144. D. B. Komaroff, "Symptoms and Signs of Chronic Fatigue Syndrome," *Reviews of Infectious Diseases* 13, suppl. (1991): S8–11.

145. D. Buchwald et al., "A Chronic Illness Characterized by Fatigue, Neurological and Immunological Disorders, and Active Human Herpesvirus Type 6 Infection," *Annals of Internal Medicine* 116 (1992): 103–13.

146. A. B. Adolphe, "Chronic Fatigue Syndrome: Possible Effective Treatment with Nifedipine," *American Journal of Medicine* 85 (1988): 892.

147. Y. Hokama and J. L. R. Y. Hokama, "*In Vitro* Inhibition of Platelet Aggregation

with Low Dalton Compounds from Aqueous Dialysates of Edible Fungi," *Research Communications in Chemical Pathology and Pharmacology* 31 (1981): 177–80.

148. K. Takashima et al., "The Hypocholesterolemic Action of Eritadenine in the Rat," *Atherosclerosis* 17 (1973): 491–502.

149. T. Saitoh, "Effect of Eritadenine on Lipids in Hepatic Bile," in *Mushroom Science IX* (Part I), proceedings of the Ninth International Scientific Congress on the Cultivation of Edible Fungi, Tokyo, 1974 (Kiryu, Japan: Mushroom Research Institute, 1976), 469–76.

150. H. Takazawa et al., "An Antiviral Compound from 'Shiitake' (*Lentinus edodes*)," *Yakugaku Zasshi* 102 (1982): 489–91.

151. M. Togami et al., "Studies on Basidiomycetes. I. Antitumor Polysaccharides from Bagasse Medium on Which Mycelia of *Lentinus edodes* (Berk.) Sing. Had Been Grown," *Chemical and Pharmaceutical Bulletin* 30 (1982): 1134–40.

152. K. H. Jeune et al., "Studies on Lectins from Korean Higher Fungi. IV. A Mitogenic Lectin from the Mushroom *Lentinus edodes*," *Planta Medica* 56 (1990): 592 (poster).

153. G. Chihara et al., "Fractionation and Purification of the Polysaccharides with Marked Antitumor Activity, Especially Lentinan, from *Lentinus edodes* (Berk.) Sing. (An Edible Mushroom)," *Cancer Research* 30 (1970): 2776–81.

154. T. Aoki, "Lentinan," in *Immune Modulation Agents and Their Mechanisms*, eds., R. L. Fenishel and M. A. Chirgis (New York and Basel: Marcel Dekker, 1984), 63–77.

155. G. Chihara et al., "Antitumor and Metastasis-Inhibitory Activities of Lentinan As an Immunomodulator: An Overview," *Cancer Detection and Prevention Supplement* 1 (1987): 423–43.

156. Y. Kaneko et al., "Activity of Lentinan Against Cancer and AIDS," *International Journal of Immunotherapy* 5 (1989): 203–13.

157. See note 9 above.

158. T. Suzuki and T. Ikegawa, "Anticancer Substance, Emitanin," in *Chemical Abstracts* 87 (1977): 539 (C.A. 87:199155d).

159. K. Sorimachi et al., "Anti-viral Activity of Water-solubilized Lignin Derivatives *in Vitro*," *Agricultural and Biological Chemistry* 54 (1990): 1337–39.

160. H. Suzuki et al., "Structural Characterization of the Immunoactive and Antiviral Water-solubilized Lignin in an Extract of the Culture Medium of *Lentinus edodes* Mycelia (LEM)," *Agricultural and Biological Chemistry* 54 (1990): 479–87.

161. F. Suzuki et al., "Antiviral and Interferon-Inducing Activities of a New Peptidomannan, KS-2, Extracted from Culture Mycelia of *Lentinus edodes*," *Journal of Antibiotics* 32 (1979): 1336–45.

162. T. Fujii et al., "Isolation and Characterization of a New Antitumor Polysaccharide, KS-2, Extracted from Culture Mycelia of *Lentinus edodes*," *Journal of Antibiotics* 31 (1978): 1079–90.

163. N. Ishida et al., "Antitumor Agent KS-2-B," *U.K. Patent Application* GB 2 023 131 A, Dec. 28, 1979.

164. M. Takehara et al., "Antiviral and Antitumor Activities of Certain Double-Stranded Polyribonucleotides," *ICRM Annals* 3 (1983): 81–88.

165. M. Takehara et al., "Antiviral Activity of Virus-Like Particles from *Lentinus edodes* (Shiitake)," *Archives of Virology* 59 (1979): 269–74.

166. Y. Yamamura and K. W. Cochran, "A Selective Inhibitor of Myxoviruses from Shii-ta-ke (*Lentinus edodes*)," in *Mushroom Science IX* (Part I), proceedings of the Ninth International Scientific Congress on the Cultivation of Edible Fungi, Tokyo, 1974 (Kiryu, Japan: Mushroom Research Institute, 1976), 495–507.

167. N. Kobayashi et al., "Purification and Chemical Properties of an Inhibitor of Plant Virus Infection from Fruiting Bodies of *Lentinus edodes*," *Agricultural and Biological Chemistry* 51 (1987): 883–90.

168. Y. Kurashima et al., "Marked Formation of Thiazolidine-4-carboxylic Acid, an Effective Nitrite Trapping Agent *in Vivo*, on Boiling of Dried Shiitake Mushroom (*Lentinus edodes*)," *Journal of Agriculture and Food Chemistry* 38 (1990): 1945–49.

Index